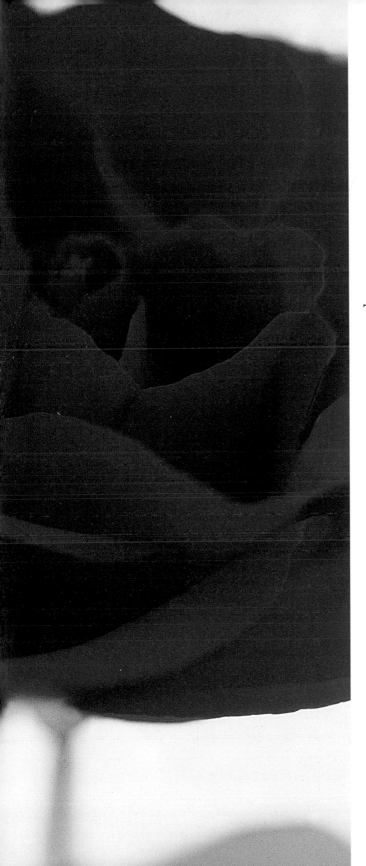

AYURVEDA

The ancient Indian medical system,
focusing on the prevention
of disease through diet,
lifestyle and herbalism

GOPI WARRIER

with a team of doctors from the Ayurvedic
Charitable Hospital and the Ayurveda College

CARLTON
BOOKS

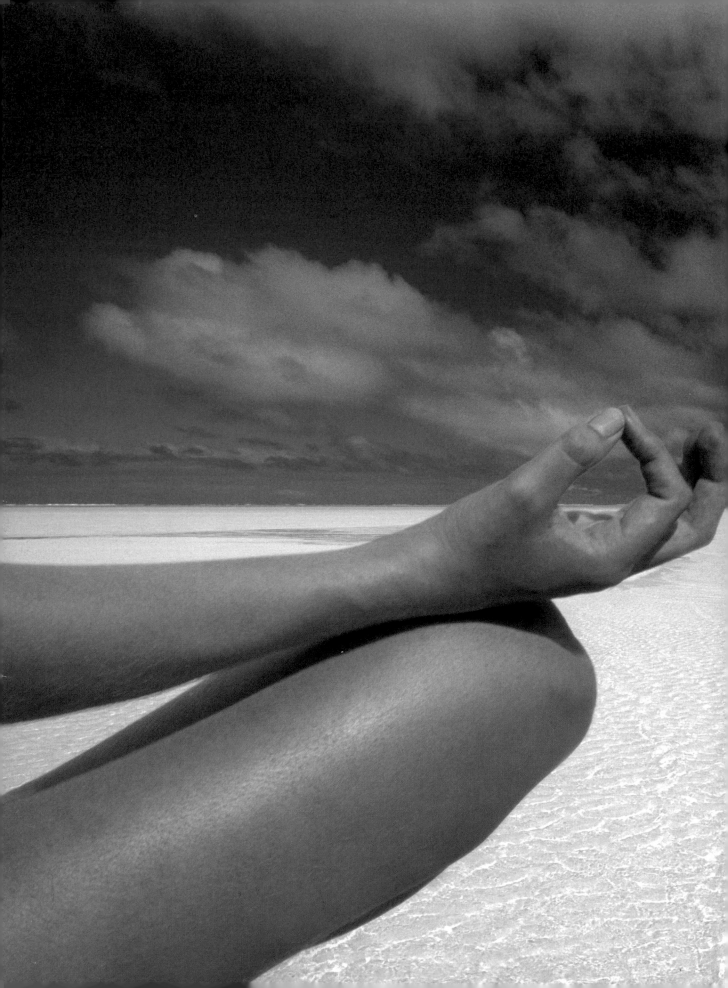

AYURVEDA

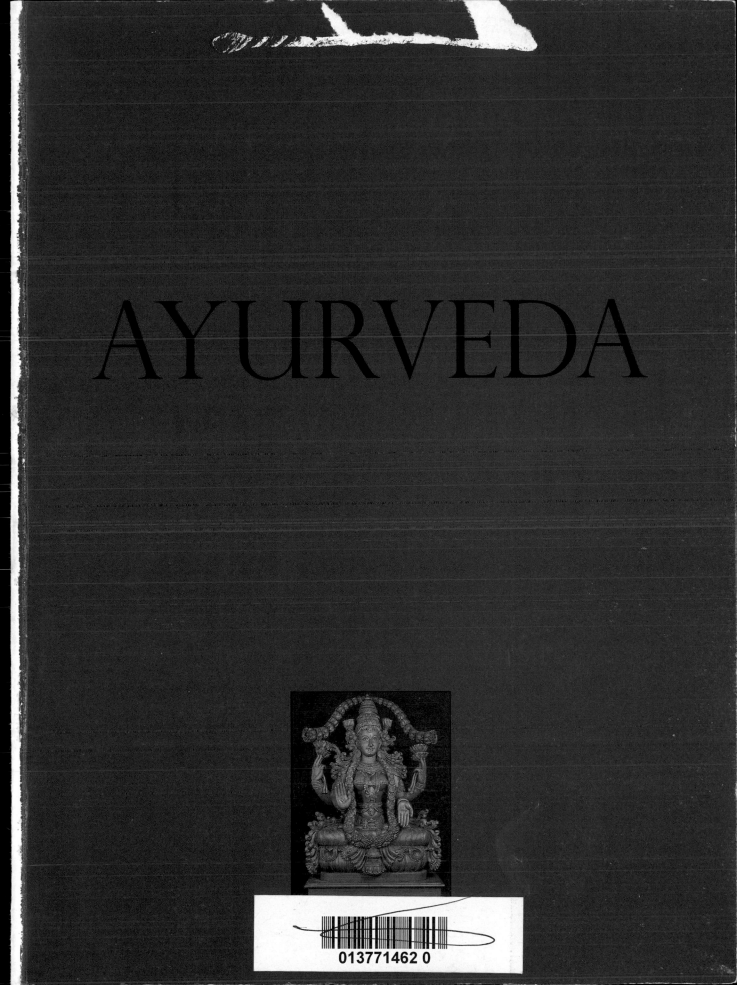

THIS IS A CARLTON BOOK

Text copyright © 2002 Gopi Warrier
Design, special photography and illustrations
copyright © Carlton Books Limited 2002

This edition published in 2013 by
Carlton Books Limited
20 Mortimer Street
London W1T 3JW

10 9 8 7 6 5 4 3 2 1

ISBN: 978-1-78097-262-6

Printed and bound in Dubai

The authors and publisher have made every
effort to ensure that all information is correct
and up to date at the time of publication.
Neither the authors nor the publisher can accept
responsibility for any accident, injury or damage
that results from using the ideas, information or
advice offered in this book.

All who seek Ayurvedic treatment are warned
that they should avoid consultation with therapist
who do not have a minimum of a recognized
university degree in Ayurveda as this could
endanger their health.

contents

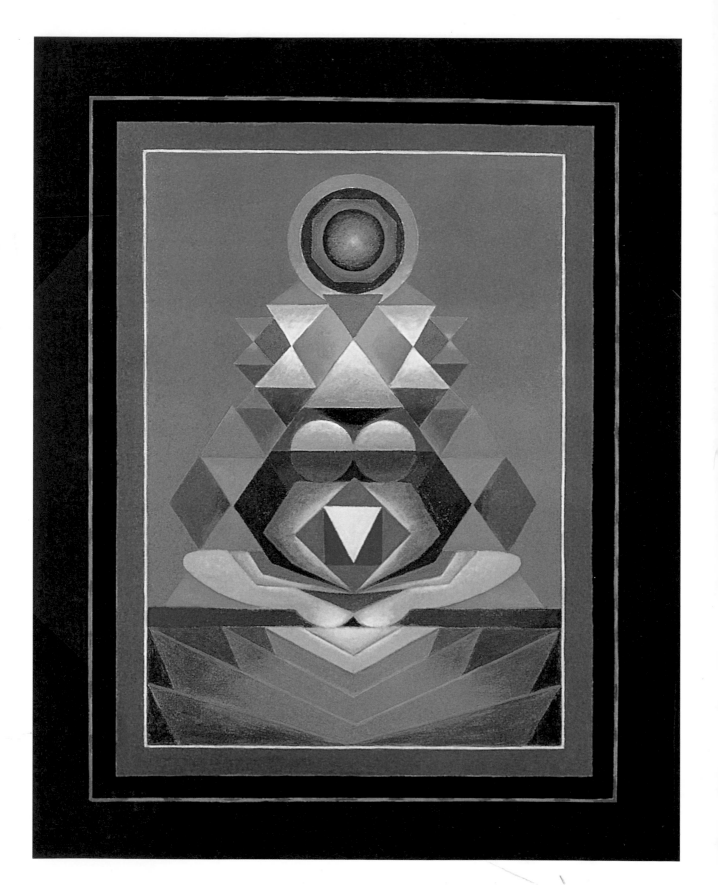

Introduction

Originating from the Indus Valley in India, ayurveda is the oldest medical practice in the world, dating back to around 3500 BC. Today, this ancient system of treatment is attracting growing interest and wider use all over the world. Its aim is to diagnose by evaluating both the body and the mind. Thus, with the appropriate treatment, people can lead healthy and fulfilling lives. A holistic system consisting of diet, yoga, massage, detoxification, herbal medicine and meditation, ayurveda improves not only your health, but also your wellbeing, behaviour and state of mind. It has been used for centuries to treat many diseases, including paralysis, diabetes, mental illnesses, rheumatoid arthritis and respiratory diseases, as well as minor ailments, disease prevention and rejuvenation.

Ayurveda treats your mind, body and spirit, and relieves symptoms of disease. Moreover, it can be used on a long-term basis with no ill effect and helps to prevent illness, rather than simply waiting to cure it. Prevention is a key tenet in ayurveda.

According to ayurveda, the universe and each individual within it are composed of five elements, called the *panchamahabhutas*, and three vital energies, called the doshas. The five elements are air, fire, water, earth and space; the three doshas are *vata*, *kapha* and *pitta*. An imbalance in the doshas will bring about illness and disease. Ayurveda is utilized to restore equilibrium between the three doshas and to obtain perfect health.

left **COSMIC BEING IN MEDITATION, BY G SANTOSH**

Each one of us is made up of the three doshas in differing proportions, and the individual's distinct composition is dependent upon the state of the parents' doshas at the time of conception. This physical constitution, or *prakruti*, remains constant for the whole of a person's life.

We can consist of one type of dosha or a combination, such as vata-kapha or pitta-vata. The ayurvedic practitioner tries to determine each patient's constitution and provide the appropriate treatment. This may involve a change in your diet and lifestyle, as well as ayurvedic therapy, ayurvedic medicine or herbal treatments, or rejuvenation therapy.

The three doshas play a very important role in ayurveda. Each one has its own input. Vata is related to the body's energy and nervous system, pitta is related to temperature, heat and the biochemical processes in the body, and kapha is related to the maintenance of the skeletal system, strength and formation of the body.

Furthermore, the three doshas greatly affect the characteristics and features of a person. They determine our basic nature, the colour of our hair, the appearance of our skin, our tone of voice, body frame and appetite, for example. While some people prefer certain foods, others cannot tolerate them; this is due to the different constitution of each individual.

Learning to harness this knowledge in all its complexity, with the help of a properly qualified ayurvedic practitioner, can bring you untold benefits in terms of living a longer, happier and healthier life.

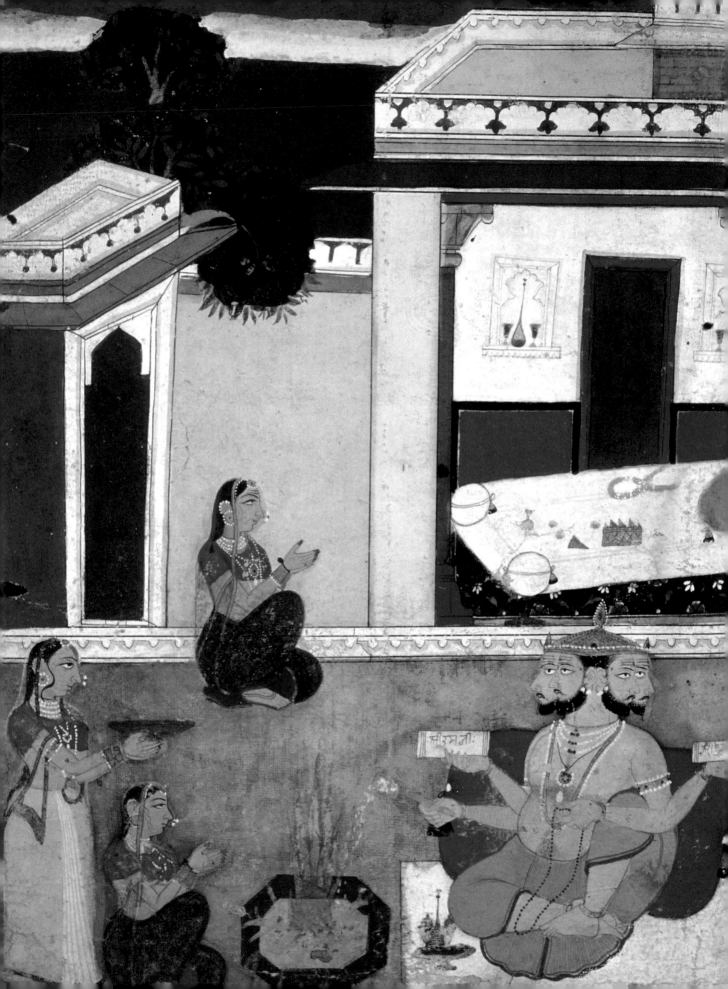

1 the history of ayurveda

Ayurvedic mythology

Ayurveda is a Sanskrit word meaning the knowledge or science of life. As a collective medical system, it predates all others. The first known recorded evidence of the medicinal properties of plants, minerals and metals dates back to around 4500 BC. This is the approximate time when the first of the Vedas or sciences, the *Rig Veda*, was written. Centuries later, when the Vedic text *Atharvaveda* was written (c 1500–1000 BC), one finds the treatment of disease, with particular emphasis on mantras, penances, amulets, sacred rituals and herbal medicines.

Ayurveda is the very foundation of ancient medical science and is considered supplementary to the *Atharvaveda*, which means 'the knowledge of the wise and the old'. The Hindu god Brahma, the creator of the universe in Hindu mythology, originated the system. Brahma then passed it on to the Aswini Kumars (physicians of the gods) and Indra, the god of weather and rain. Internal medicine was disclosed by Indra primarily to the sage Atreya Punarvasu, and this formed the classical *Charaka* tradition of ayurvedic general medicine. Surgery was divulged by Indra to Divodasa, the king of Kashi, who is an incarnation of divine Dhanvantari, the god of ayurveda. This ultimately formed the classical *Sushruta* tradition of ayurvedic surgery and medicine (see the birth of ayurveda, page 10). The knowledge was passed on to the sages, from where it was disseminated and promoted among the people over the following generations.

The influence of ayurveda can be seen quite clearly in traditional Chinese medicine, as well as in Tibetan medicine and the traditional healing systems of other Buddhist countries, such as Sri Lanka and Burma.

left **AN OFFERING IS MADE TO THE HINDU GOD, BRAHMA, THE CREATOR OF THE UNIVERSE IN HINDU MYTHOLOGY. THE SYSTEM OF AYURVEDA IS BELIEVED TO HAVE ORIGINATED WITH BRAHMA**

In ancient times, both the gods and demons – debilitated by old age and illness – asked Vishnu, the god of preservation, how to regain their strength and health. Lord Vishnu told them that the only way to achieve perfect health was to invoke Dhanvantari, the god of ayurveda. Vishnu explained that they must then select a number of species of herb and throw them into the ocean. Next, using a mountain as the churning rod, the gods and the demons had to churn the ocean. Vishnu would form the base of the mountain, taking the form of a tortoise, while the powerful serpent Vasuki would be the churning rope. The gods and the demons followed Vishnu's instructions. The selected herbs were thrown into the sea and the demons and gods began to churn. Unfortunately, something went wrong, as the process was started without prayers to Lord Ganapathy, the elephant god who removes all obstacles. The gods and demons were all unprotected. The serpent Vasuki warned that he would soon be forced to spit out his poison, as he was exhausted. It was so venomous, however, that it would kill all living beings if it fell upon the Earth.

The gods asked Shiva, the compassionate one who is regarded as both destroyer and restorer, to swallow the poison, as only he could withstand the venom. Lord Shiva agreed, but his wife, Parvati, ran to Shiva and squeezed his neck as tightly as she could to prevent the poison from flowing down into his body, so concerned was she about his safety. The poison remained in Shiva's throat, colouring his neck blue. Vishnu realized that the reason this problem had arisen was that the proper preparations had not been made, and he instructed all the assembled gods and demons to pray to Ganapathy, the elephant god, for protection. After this, they would be able to recommence the churning.

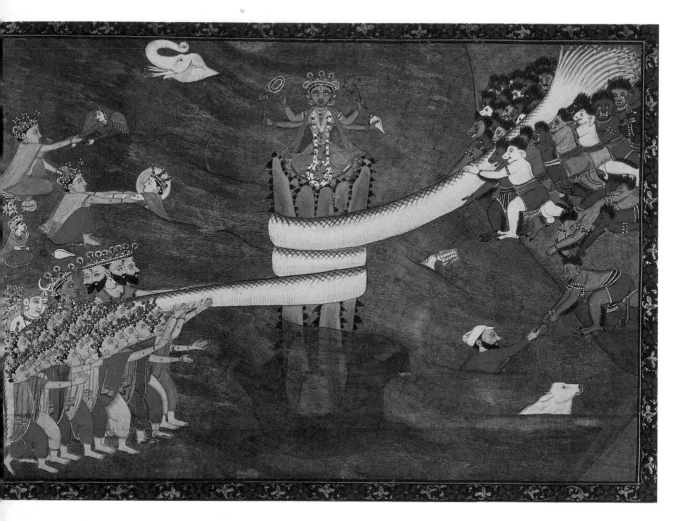

above **THE GODS AND THE DEMONS CHURN THE OCEAN UNDER THE GUIDANCE OF LORD VISHNU, IN ORDER TO INVOKE DHANVANTARI, THE GOD OF AYURVEDA, WHO WOULD RESTORE THEM TO THEIR FORMER STATE OF GOOD HEALTH AND STRENGTH**

Once this was done and the churning began again, all sorts of gems, beautiful trees and elephants came out of the ocean, including Lakshmi, the goddess of wealth. Finally, Dhanvantari emerged from the ocean with the elixir of life; however, before the gods could greet him, the elixir was snatched from his hands by the demons. The gods again asked Vishnu for help, and this time he adopted the form of a seductive angel and persuaded the demons to close their eyes while they drank the elixir. As soon as their eyes were closed, Vishnu took the elixir and returned it to the gods, who consumed it quickly to regain their radiance.

This story demonstrates the great effort required to restore the ecological balance of Earth and protect its resources and biodiversity, which should be distributed on an equal and fair basis to all.

The birth of ayurveda

The history of ayurveda dates back to around 4000 BC. Ayurvedic texts refer to Maharishi Bharadwaja as being instrumental in compiling information on the science and presenting it as an independent branch of medicine. The history of ayurvedic medicine can be broadly placed into two periods: the classical text period from about the second century BC, and the compilation period from the early centuries AD.

In the classical era, the two most important reference texts on ayurvedic medicine and surgery were composed. The *Charaka Samhita* on medicine was written by Charaka, and the *Sushruta Samhita* on surgery written by Sushruta. Both were renowned ayurvedic practitioners. The *Charaka Samhita*, which is considered sacred, consists of 150 chapters on specific topics. It contains detailed classification and nomenclature of diseases, their definition, their causes, early features, symptoms, prognosis and treatment, including the selection and administration of drugs, and the importance of a healthy diet and general practices. According to Charaka, ayurvedic medicine consists of eight branches:

- Internal medicine and therapeutics
- Specific organ diseases – eye, ear, nose, throat
- Surgery
- Toxicology
- Psychiatry
- Paediatrics
- Rejuvenation
- Virilification – the use of aphrodisiacs and fertility-boosting agents to improve sexual function and generative tissues

The contents of the *Sushruta Samhita* are similar to that of the *Charaka Samhita*, but with special emphasis on surgery. Sushruta considered surgery to be the best among the therapies, as it can produce instantaneous relief by means of instruments and appliances. The treatise discusses various types of inflammations, wounds, burns and fractures. Many major operations for intestinal obstructions, bladder stones, amputation, extraction of foreign bodies, and plastic surgery such as rhinoplasty, are described.

Another important ayurvedic text is the *Ashtanga Samgraha*, written by Vagbhatta, who worked in the medical school at the Nalanda University in the seventh century BC. Vagbhatta has very succinctly discussed the work of Charaka and Sushruta, and at the same time given a lot of original views on the management of many different diseases.

In India, numerous other medicinal texts have been compiled on ayurveda throughout the centuries, with the influence from various other systems of medicine that came along with the invasions of the Indian subcontinent first by the Greeks, then the Arabs and finally the British. Over the years, a vast pharmacopoeia has been added to this highly complex system of knowledge, one that is fast expanding as a scientific tradition with proven safety and efficacy.

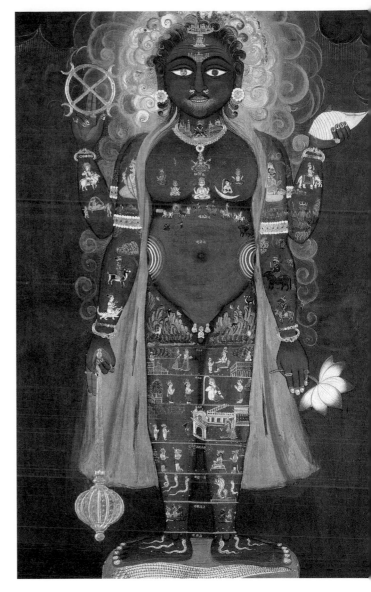

above right **VISHNU, THE GOD OF PRESERVATION, WHO EXPLAINED TO THE GODS AND DEMONS HOW TO INVOKE DHANVANTARI**
right **ANCIENT AYURVEDIC TEXT ON PALM LEAF,** c AD 800

Ayurveda and the environment

Our sense of wellbeing depends very much on maintaining the equilibrium of the three doshas (see pages 20–7 and 44–5) and achieving a balance between mind, body and spirit. The ancient wisdom of ayurveda places just as much emphasis on leading a lifestyle that is in harmony with the environment.

The unprecedented increase in the scale and intensity of human activity, combined with population growth, has resulted in a situation where humankind's 'ecological footprint' has been stamped over much of the planet and is threatening key resources on which we and other living species depend. Technological advances, industrialization and urbanization have led to the production of global pollutants and consumption of non-renewable resources. As a result, the over-use of agricultural chemicals, the contamination of food products and the pollution of soil and water are growing problems. More recently, public concerns about animal husbandry practices in the UK and many European countries have been heightened in the wake of the widespread incidence of bovine spongiform encephalopathy (BSE), salmonellosis, and the foot-and-mouth epidemic.

The classical ayurvedic text *Charaka Samhita*, dated second century BC, states unequivocally that air, water, land and the seasons are indispensable for life. Degrading or destroying these environmental factors leads to the manifestation of disease. The knock-on effect of pollution of natural resources is graphically described in a chapter of the *Charaka Samhita* devoted to the specific characteristics of epidemics:

**... because of the disappearance of righteous acts ... seasons are impaired.
Consequently, either there is no rainfall in time or there is no rainfall at all;
Or there is an abnormality in the rainfall;
Air does not blow properly;
There is abnormality in the earth, water (reservoirs) dries up;
Drugs lose their normal attributes and are impaired.
Then there is impairment of the country because of the impairment of food and drink.**

Charaka Samhita, **Vimanasthana**

Ayurveda emphasizes that our personal health can be maintained by following a health-promoting daily and seasonal regimen, through the proper application of the intellect and discrimination between wholesome and unwholesome thoughts, words and deeds. The same principles form the base of ayurveda's approach to the protection of the environment. Truthfulness, compassion for living beings, charity, adoption of preventive measures and self-control are identified as some of the attributes needed to prevent epidemics and to safeguard natural resources which sustain life.

In ayurveda, plants and herbs are recognized as some of the greatest gifts of nature to humankind. Like all living creatures, they are a microcosm of the universe and a combination of the elemental qualities of earth, water, fire, air and ether (space). Their potency as food and medicines is largely determined by the quality of their habitat, cultivation methods, the season in which they are harvested, storage methods and processing. The ideal herbal plant or drug is one which is grown in an auspicious place and collected on an auspicious day after due deference is paid by someone who follows a *satvic*, or noble and strong, way of life. The respect accorded to plants goes beyond ayurveda as a system of healthcare, however, to its roots in Hindu culture and tradition.

Many plants are associated with particular Hindu deities. Bilwa leaves (*Aegle marmelos Corr.*) are offered in the worship of Shiva, the destroyer, and the roots, bark and fruits of the tree are used in different formulations for a range of conditions, including diabetes mellitus, chronic diarrhoea, insomnia and anxiety neurosis. This tree grows wild all over the sub-Himalayan forests and in many other parts of India, and it is specially cultivated and tended in the vicinity of Shiva temples.

Holy basil (*Ocimum sanctum Linn.*), known as *tuli* in Sanskrit, is another sacred plant, one which is chiefly associated with the worship of Vishnu. Holy basil is grown in the courtyard of many Hindu homes and is worshipped daily as part of the household's religious rituals. The folk traditions of India recognize the powerful therapeutic potential of basil, particularly for the common cold and cough, skin infections and indigestion. The classical ayurvedic pharmacopoeia includes a number of formulations in which various parts of the plant are a major ingredient.

Haritaki (*Terminalia chebula Retz.*) is believed to have originated from a drop of nectar which fell to the ground when Indra, the Lord of the gods, was partaking of it, while the Buddha is believed to have attained enlightenment while meditating under a pippali, or long pepper, tree (*Piper longum Linn.*).

As various international conventions are held to discuss climate change, deforestation and depletion of the ozone layer by industrially produced chlorofluoro-carbons (CFCs), and the World Health Organization stresses the urgent need to create a sustainable healthy environment, the advice given in the ayurvedic texts seems to have a particular resonance.

Our environment is a complex amalgamation of ecosystems, each made up of a variety of species. Ensuring that we preserve and protect our environment, in accordance with the rhythms of nature, is essential. For instance, biodiversity is necessary for the long-term sustainability of the environment and indispensable to human health. For each plant that is picked for medicinal purposes, the ayurvedic practitioner is exhorted to cultivate a replacement, thereby restoring the balance in nature.

The health-promoting benefits of a constructed environment which conforms to natural principles were also recognized by the founding fathers of ayurveda. Recommendations given in the *Charaka Samhita* for building a child's nursery, a maternity home and a hospital closely follow the rules laid down by the Vedic science of architecture, *vastu shastra*. All buildings are believed to have a spiritual dimension and the quality of the soil on which a building is sited, the shape and elevation of the land, the direction in which the building faces and the materials used in its construction all have an impact on the health and general wellbeing of the occupants.

Vastu shastra, like ayurveda, takes into account the five elements – earth, water, fire, air and space – and aims to balance these in the correct proportions for prosperity and harmony. Of the eight directions, the east and the north are considered particularly important and buildings should ideally face one of these directions. Construction should commence only after ritual consecration of the land and purification rituals must be performed before occupation,.

The principles of the Vedic science of architecture have a universal application. The essence of this classical science is believed to have spread eastwards along with Buddhism, much like ayurveda itself. Feng shui, the Chinese approach to creating a harmonious living and working environment, which has become increasingly popular in the West, incorporates many of the concepts of *vastu shastra*.

below **AYURVEDA ADVOCATES A LIFESTYLE THAT PROTECTS THE EARTH'S RESOURCES AND IS IN HARMONY WITH THE ENVIRONMENT**

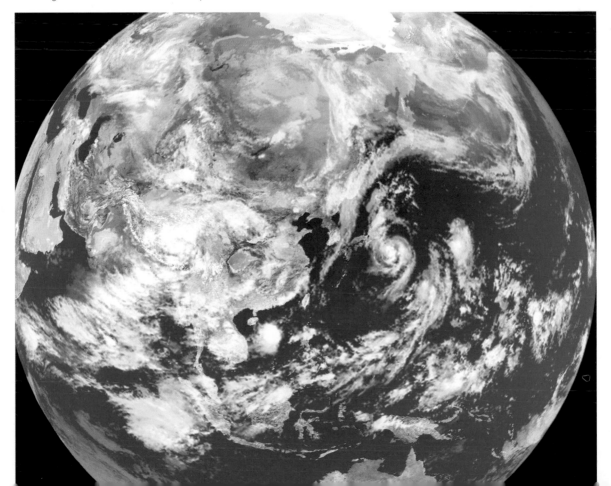

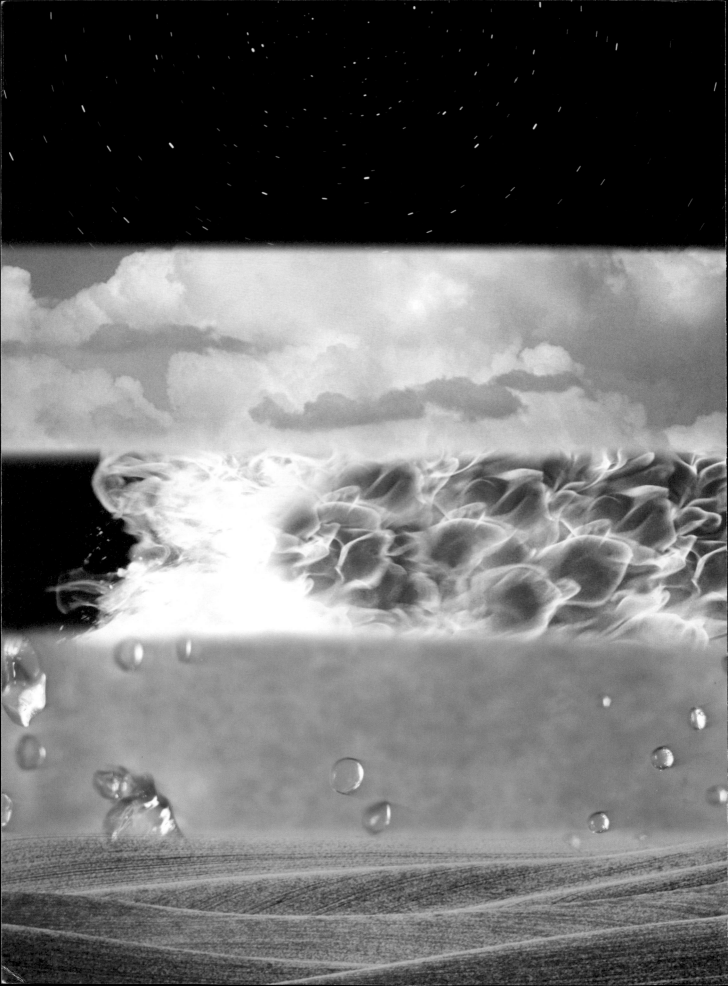

2 the philosophy of ayurveda

Ayurveda aims to relieve symptoms, prevent illness and help you lead and maintain a healthy lifestyle. So, how does it work? In ayurveda, there is an evaluation of the entire body and mind – it aims to heal the whole patient, rather than simply treat the disease in isolation. It is a holistic system that combines medication, diet, yoga, massage, detoxification and the use of herbs and oils to gain optimum health. Although ayurveda can be and is used to treat various diseases and illnesses, such as asthma, stress, constipation and rheumatoid arthritis, at its very foundation lies the importance of preventing long-term illness, rather than waiting for a disorder to manifest itself. In ayurvedic medicine it is believed that everything within the universe, including us, is composed of the five elements – air, fire, water, earth and space – and the three doshas – vata, pitta and kapha. The doshas are affected by the five elements and, in turn, perfect health is only achieved when each of the three doshas is in equilibrium within us.

The five elements

Ayurveda draws its fundamental concepts and theories from various Hindu schools of philosophy, such as Samkhya, Yoga and Nyaya. The underlying premise of all these philosophical schools is that the entire universe is made up of five basic elements, or *panchamahabhutas*, in various proportions.

Breaking the word *panchamahabhutas* into its elements, *pancha* means five; *maha* means great, mighty, strong and abundant; and *bhuta* means

left **IN AYURVEDA, EVERYTHING WITHIN THE UNIVERSE IS SAID TO BE MADE UP OF A COMBINATION OF THE FIVE ELEMENTS OF EARTH, WATER, FIRE, AIR AND SPACE. HEALTH AND WELLBEING ARE CONSIDERED TO BE A PERFECT BALANCE OF THESE**

being or creature. The theory of *panchamahabhutas* developed in the post-Vedic period from about 500 BC, particularly during the time when the *Upanishads*, the main spiritual teachings of ancient India, were written.

The five elements are:

- Earth
- Water
- Fire (energy)
- Air
- Space (ether)

So why are there only considered to be five elements? Human beings are endowed with five senses: hearing, touch, sight, taste and smell. It is through these senses that we perceive the outside world. They are our link with the physical world around us. Each sense has its own particular role to play. For instance, the sense of hearing can appreciate only the quality of sound. Touch, colour, taste, smell and sound are the five sense objects corresponding to our five senses. These are special *gunas*, or properties, and as such cannot exist independently, but must have some receptacle. In this way, we get five receptacles – the five elements.

All matter is a mixture of the five elements. Sushruta, one of the greatest authorities on ayurveda, said: 'All substances are derived from a combination of the five bhutas, and the predominance of any one of these in a particular substance determines its character, and so we say, this is watery, this is fiery, etc.'

The five elements in nature each try to dominate over one another, for example, wind or storm (air) may extinguish fire, cause the evaporation of water or destroy buildings. Fire may heat the air, evaporate liquids and burn solids. Water exerts its cooling effect on air, extinguishes fire and submerges earth. Earth,

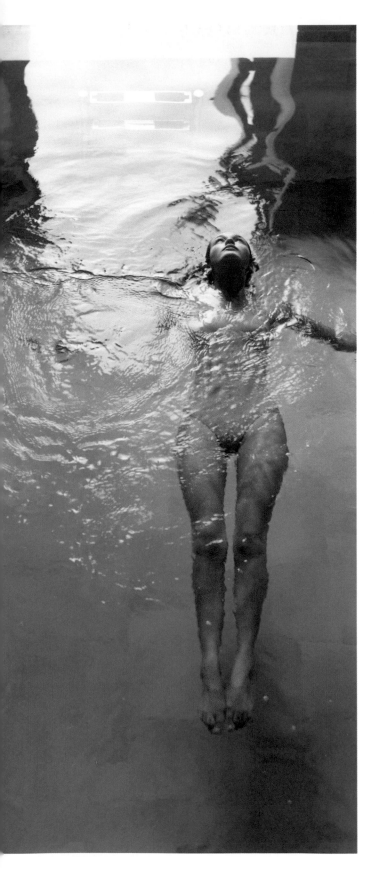

left WATER IS A VITAL CONSTITUENT OF THE HUMAN BODY. IT HELPS TO MAINTAIN THE BALANCE OF FLUIDS WITHIN EACH OF US AND IS FOUND IN PLASMA, BLOOD, SALIVA, DIGESTIVE JUICES, MUCOUS MEMBRANES AND CYTOPLASM

or solids, can hinder the wind, reduce the heat of fire and inhibit the cooling effect of water. The five elements, when in balance and functioning normally, are essential for sustaining life. These same five elements, when out of balance or exaggerated, can cause discomfort and even destroy life.

The human body, too, is composed of the five basic elements of earth, water, fire, air and space. They are linked to all aspects of our bodies (see the table opposite). After conception, space provides the fertilized ovum with room to grow; air brings about cell division; fire, or energy, helps in the transformation and digestion of nutrients; water maintains the balance of fluids such as blood, plasma and digestive juices within the body; and earth provides food for growth and keeps the cell mass together. After death, the body decomposes and merges with the same five basic elements.

Health and wellbeing can be defined as a state of perfect balance between the five basic elements, both in quantity and quality. Disease results from a change in the composition or balance of the elements, whether it be quantitatively, qualitatively or both. For example, your body will become dehydrated if the water element is diminished, while replacing fluids helps your body to rehydrate.

The food which nourishes our bodies is also derived from the five elements in various proportions. For example, rice and wheat predominate in the earth element, while milk and fruit juices are part of the water element. Pulses increase the production of gases in the body, representing the element of air. Popcorn contains much more space than the corn from which it is derived, therefore its dominant element is space, while chillies and spices represent the element of fire, or energy.

The constituents of ayurvedic drugs and medicines are also based on the five elements. If your agni (digestive fire, or metabolism) is weak or sluggish, you should use spices which are fiery in nature. If you are suffering from oedema or swelling, you should avoid salt because of its role in the retention of water.

From these examples, it is easy to see the intricate link between the theory of the five elements and ayurvedic medicine and healthcare.

The properties and functions of the five elements

	EARTH	WATER	FIRE	AIR	SPACE
PROPERTIES	Heavy	Heavy	Light,	Light	Light
	Rough	Fluid	Rough/sharp	Rough	Smooth
	Hard	Soft	Clear	Clear	Soft
	Slow, inactive	Inactive	Minute	Minute	Inactive
	Steady, firm	Slimy	Atomic	Atomic	Clear
					Minute
	Neither hot	Cold	Hot	Neither hot	Neither hot
	nor cold			nor cold	nor cold
	Clear	Dense	Dry	Active movement	
	Dense	Large molecules	Luminous		
	Large, bulky	Viscous	Active spread		Separation
		Wet, moving in	High speed		Differentiation
		the direction			
		of gravity			
MOVEMENT	Downwards	Downwards	Upwards	Centrifugal	Absent
TASTE					
Predominant	Sweet	Sweet	Pungent	Astringent	None
Associated	Slightly	Slightly	Slightly sour	Slightly bitter	
	astringent	astringent	and salty		
SENSE					
Special sense	Smell	Taste	Vision	Touch	Sound
Sense organ	Nose	Tongue	Eye	Skin	Ear
BODY					
Body	All organs in	All fluids in	All over the	All body	All body
	the body	the body	body – manifest	activities	activities
	Strength/firmness		or unmanifest	Gases	
Parts of the body	Nails	Body fluids	Pitta	Lungs and	Large spaces
	Bones	Blood	Heat	intestines	in the body –
	Tendons	Fatty tissue	Lustre	All movements	for example,
	Teeth	Kapha, pitta		in the body –	thorax, abdomen
	Muscles	Urine		for example,	All body
	Skin	Stools		muscles, cells	passages and
	Hair	Perspiration			cavities – for
	Stools	Saliva			example, nostrils,
	Spinal cord	Semen			mouth
DIET	Rice, wheat	Milk	Spices – for	Various gases	Popcorn
	Mineral salt	Fruits	example, ginger,	(air, oxygen)	Guduchi
	Carrot		pepper,		(*Tinosporia*
	Beets		asafoetida (hing),		*cordifolia Miers.*)
	Shatavari		chitrak (*Plumbago*		
	(*Asparagus*		*zeylanica Linn.*)		
	racemosus Willd.)		Garlic		

The five elements are present in all aspects of our bodies and our lives. They govern our body's tissues, waste products and our minds. Their active properties are made up from the 20 qualities of ayurveda (see page 36) and are also linked to pharmachological actions within our bodies, taste and the seasons.

The five elements, body tissues & waste products

BODY TISSUE (DHATU)	PREDOMINANT ELEMENT
Lymph (rasa)	Water
Blood (rakta)	Water + fire
Muscular tissue (mansa)	Earth
Fatty tissue (meda)	Water + earth
Bony tissue (asthi)	Earth + air
Nervous tissue and bone marrow (maija)	Water
Semen/reproductive tissue (shukra)	Water

SUBTISSUE	
Milk (stanya)	Water
Menstrual discharge (raja)	Fire

WASTE PRODUCT (MALA)	
Urine (mootram)	Water + fire
Faeces (pureesha)	Water + earth
Expired air (swasa)	Earth + air
Perspiration (sweda)	Water

The five elements & active properties

ACTIVE PROPERTY	ELEMENT
Cold	Earth + water
Hot	Fire
Viscous, unctuous	Water
Dry	Air
Heavy	Earth + water
Light	Fire + space + air
Soft	Water + space
Sharp	Fire

The five elements & the mind

ELEMENT	MENTAL QUALITY (GUNA)
Space	Satvic (noble and strong)
Air	Rajas (human and egotistical)
Fire (energy)	Satvic + rajas
Water	Satvic + tamas
Earth	Tamas (human and vulnerable)

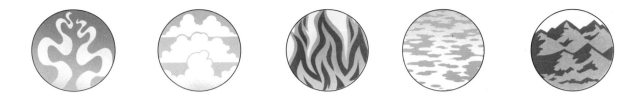

The five elements & taste

CAUSATIVE ELEMENTS	TASTE
Earth + water	Sweet
Earth + fire	Sour
Water + fire	Sour
Water + fire	Salty
Air + fire	Pungent
Air + space	Bitter
Air + earth	Astringent

The five elements, the seasons & taste

SEASON	PREDOMINANT ELEMENT	PREDOMINANT TASTE
Late winter (*Shishir*)	Air + space	Bitter
Spring (*Vasant*)	Air + earth	Astringent
Summer (*Greeshma*)	Air + fire	Pungent
Monsoon (*Varsha*)	Earth + fire	Sour
Autumn (*Sharad*)	Water + fire	Salty
Early winter (*Hemant*)	Earth + water	Sweet

The five elements & pharmacological actions

SITE OF ACTION	BASIC ELEMENT RESPONSIBLE FOR ACTION
Lower parts of body	Earth, water
Upper parts of body	Fire + air
Both upper and lower parts	Fire + air

PHARMACOLOGICAL ACTION	
Astringent	Earth, air
Soothing and stimulating	Air, water, earth
Digestive juices	Water, fire
Nourishing	Earth, water
Cooling	Water
Producing oedema (swelling)	Earth, water
Relieving oedema	Space + air
Digestion	Fire
Healing of wounds	Earth, water, air

The five elements & the three doshas

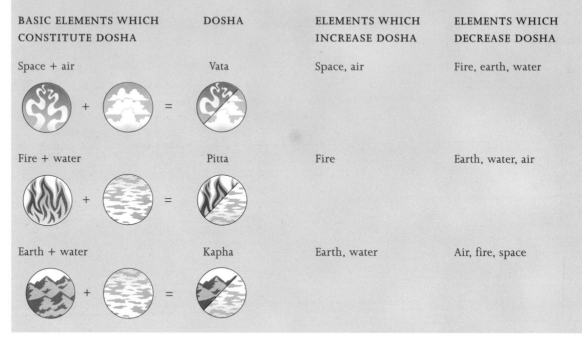

BASIC ELEMENTS WHICH CONSTITUTE DOSHA	DOSHA	ELEMENTS WHICH INCREASE DOSHA	ELEMENTS WHICH DECREASE DOSHA
Space + air	Vata	Space, air	Fire, earth, water
Fire + water	Pitta	Fire	Earth, water, air
Earth + water	Kapha	Earth, water	Air, fire, space

The three doshas

The theory of the three doshas is unique to ayurveda. While the theory of the five elements helps us to understand the universe, the concept of the three doshas helps us to understand the human body, its structure and its function. It gives us a better understanding of our biological nature. If the five elements of air, fire, water, space and earth are the basic elements of the universe, the three doshas are the basic biological molecules which constitute all living creatures from microbe to human.

Vata, pitta and kapha together form the three doshas. They are considered the basic pillars of our bodies, our vital energies. The terms vata, pitta and kapha (or sleshma) are derived respectively from the Sanskrit roots *va*, meaning to move or excite; *tap*, meaning to heat; and *slis*, meaning to embrace. From this, we can infer that the natural attribute of vata is motion, that of pitta is heat and that of kapha is union, integration or cohesion. These biological molecules have acquired a specific character from the elements that rule them. The elements of air and space rule the formation of vata, fire and water rule pitta, and earth and water rule kapha. Thus vata possesses the mobility of air and space, pitta displays the energy of fire, and kapha has the firmness and stability of earth plus a fluid plasticity.

All biological activities can be traced to the normal or abnormal functioning of the three doshas. Ayurveda views the balance of the three doshas as health, and the imbalance as disease. When balanced, they sustain our body and our wellbeing. Happiness and health invariably depend on the three doshas being in harmonious balance.

So why, in ayurveda, are only three doshas considered to be the basis of life processes? We have already seen that the three doshas are the outcome of the combination of the five elements. Of these, earth and space have no definite actions of their own and so are not the direct cause of any disease. It is only by the association with any one of the three other elements that these two can function. This is the reason why ayurvedic physicians postulated only three doshas – vata, pitta and kapha – corresponding to the three elements of air, fire and water.

In the same way as the external world is maintained by the forces of the air, the sun and the moon (which represents water), so the human body is maintained by the three doshas. Within the living body, vata motivates and organizes all the bodily elements, including the tissues and waste products. Pitta, with its dominant element of fire, is all about transformation. While kapha, through its qualities of preservation and conservation of energy, enables all plants and animals to grow.

What are the doshas?

The three doshas form the basis of your physical constitution, your mental capacities and your emotional make-up. Individuals can be of one type of dosha or a combination, that is, a person can be vata, pitta or kapha only, or vata-pitta, vata kapha or pitta-kapha. In fact, most people are a combination of two doshas. If an individual is vata-kapha, then it is said that these two doshas are dominant to pitta, hence there is only a small percentage of pitta. A particular combination of doshas may be ideal for one person, but cause disharmony and disease in another. The foods we eat and the lifestyle we lead will also affect the equilibrium of each of the doshas within us. As a result, ayurvedic medicine plays a very significant role in the restoration and stabilization of the doshas.

VATA is related to the body's energy and nervous system. Its main elements are air and space. Air is the dominant element, which is why vata is sometimes referred to as the air humour. Vata's qualities are light, cold, dry, rough, subtle, mobile, clear and dispersing. Vata, in its natural (normal) state, maintains the autonomous nervous system, inhalation, exhalation, movement of the body, equilibrium of tissues and acuity of the senses. Therefore, an imbalance in vata can lead to conditions such as, tiredness, insomnia and constipation. The main site of vata is the colon, where it accumulates and causes diseases and from where it can be expelled directly. People who are vata types tend to be thin, have dry skin, be highly active, speak quickly and be mentally restless. They have poor long-term memory and are emotionally frightened and insecure.

PITTA is related to temperature and the biochemical processes in the body. The main elements associated with pitta are fire and water. With fire as the dominant element, pitta is sometimes referred to as the fire humour. Pitta's qualities are light, hot, oily, sharp, liquid, sour and pungent. In its normal state, pitta is responsible for digestion, hunger, intelligence, determination and courage. An imbalance in pitta can lead to digestive problems, and result in the discoloration of faeces and urine. The main location of pitta is the small intestine. This is where pitta accumulates and the site from which it can be expelled from the body. Pitta types are of medium build, have fair skin and fair or reddish hair. They are intelligent, have a good memory and can be very competitive. Pitta types have a strong digestion and like sharp-tasting, sweet and bitter foods.

KAPHA is related to maintenance of the skeletal system, strength and formation of the body. The basic elements associated with kapha are water and earth. Water is the dominant element, and kapha is sometimes referred to as the 'water humour'. Kapha's qualities are heavy, cold, oily, slow, dense, soft, static and sweet. In the normal state, it is responsible for firmness and stability, the maintenance of body fluids, love and forgiveness. An imbalance in kapha will result in excessive mucus production, asthma, exhaustion and breathing difficulties. The site for kapha is the chest, where it accumulates and causes disease when in excess, and from where it can be directly expelled. Kapha types have a large physical frame. They are slow, caring and emotionally secure, think rationally and prefer sharp and pungent tastes.

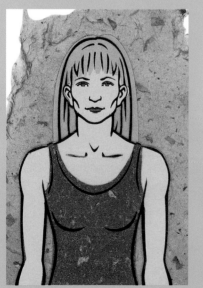

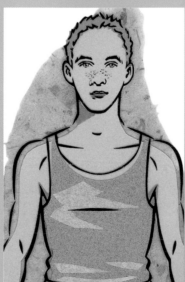

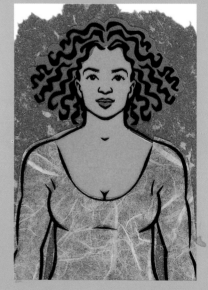

The normal seats of the doshas in the body

Each dosha is seen to reside in certain body organs or parts only. These are called their normal seats. The general view in ayurveda is that the doshas permeate the entire body and all its tissues, organs and cells. Functionally and in terms of their seats, however, the pelvic colon or lower part of the body is considered the seat of vata, the middle of the body is the seat of pitta and the chest region or upper part of the body is considered the seat of kapha.

KAPHA
Body fluids
Chest
Fatty tissues
Joints
Respiratory tract
Gastrointestinal tract
Kidneys
Head

PITTA
Digestive tract
Body fluids
Blood
Sweat
Skin
Eyes
Brain

VATA
Pelvic colon
Rectum
Bladder
Pelvis
Lower limbs
Bones
Ears
Skin

The physiological functions of the doshas

VATA

Vata is the most predominant of all the three doshas and has movements in all directions, is the quickest dosha and controls every action of our bodies. It circulates blood and body fluids, and also circulates pitta and kapha throughout our bodies.

The principal function of air (*vayu*) is to sustain and support life. That is why vayu is also referred to as *prana*, the breath of life, in ayurveda. It is also the dominant element of vata. The following are important functions of vata:

- Maintains the machinery of the body and keeps it in good order
- Initiates, organizes and controls all of the body's actions
- Regulates and guides the mind
- Operates and unites the senses – sight, hearing, smell, touch and taste
- Builds the particular structure of the different tissues and connects them together
- Generates speech
- Manifests desire and pleasure
- Kindles the internal fire
- Dries up excess moisture accumulated in the body
- Evacuates urine, faeces and other waste materials from the body
- Differentiates and forms the different channels, fine or coarse, found within the body
- Forms the different structures of the foetus

Thus, according to Charaka, the father of ayurvedic medicine, air, and thus vata, controls all effort, inhalation, exhalation, circulation, proper action of speech, mind and body, nourishment of the tissues and proper elimination of waste matter from the body. Sushruta refers to the same functions as *praspandana*, *udvahana*, *purana*, *viveka* and *dharana*.

PITTA

The principal function of pitta is to maintain the body by supplying and producing heat. This is why fire is considered the dominant element of pitta. The special functions of pitta are:

- Sight
- Digestion
- Heat (body temperature)
- Hunger, thirst and softness of the skin
- Radiance, cheerfulness and intelligence
- Colouring and pigmentation

KAPHA

The principal function of kapha is to form and preserve the body by acting as the body's watery substance, reflecting the fact that its dominant element is water. Some of the other functions are:

- Maintaining viscidity
- Binding and lubricating the joints
- Maintaining strength
- Providing solidity and strength to the body
- Sexual vigour
- Fortitude, forbearance, patience and abstinence
- Nourishment
- Immunity and resistance

The biorhythms of the doshas

The doshas show constant shifts inside the body and rhythmic fluctuations are the rule of nature. Although ideally a balanced state of the doshas is necessary for health and happiness, at no time will your doshas be in perfect equilibrium. They will always flow in tune with your age, the time of the day or night, the time of digestive function and the seasons of the year. In childhood, the kapha dosha is dominant. When you reach middle age, it is pitta that predominates, while in old age vata will be the dominant dosha.

below **THE BALANCE OF THE DOSHAS IN THE BODY SHIFTS SLIGHTLY ACCORDING TO YOUR AGE, THE TIME OF DAY OR NIGHT, THE TIME OF YEAR AND THE TIME OF DIGESTIVE FUNCTION**

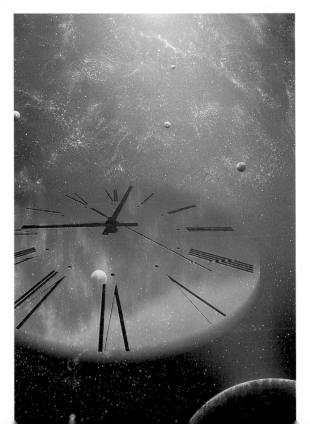

The way in which your doshas fluctuate according to the time of day follows a pattern. Kapha dosha dominates in the morning (between 6 and 10 am), pitta dominates during the afternoon (2 to 6 pm) and vata dominates in the late evening (6 pm to midnight). Similar cycles are also repeated at night. Seasonal fluctuations in the doshas also adhere to a particular pattern. In the rainy season vata dominates; during winter pitta dominates; and in early summer kapha dominates. In this way, the doshas maintain our regular biorhythms, thereby maintaining a balance within us. The biological clock is regulated by the doshic biorhythm and it is essential for sustaining life.

The relation of the three doshas to digestion, bowels, physical constitution, psychological constitution and the six tastes are given on page 27.

The doshas and Western culture

Irregular routines, long commutes, frequent travel, erratic and rushed eating habits, constant deadlines, sleep deprivation, late-night parties, smoking, alcohol, drugs and unregulated sexual activity are all too familiar characteristics of modern Western living. These are also precisely the things that will aggravate vata dosha. We are creating and living in an environment in which the stability and structure of vata is greatly threatened. If vata is aggravated or increased, it influences the other two doshas, jeopardizing their stability. Clear goals and intelligent insight into our purpose of living and our daily attitudes and habits can change all this.

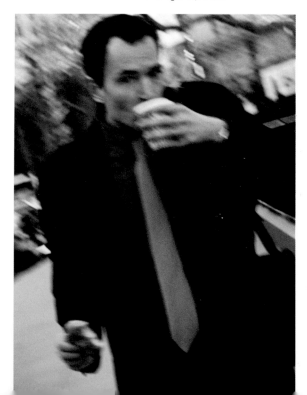

The importance of the three doshas

The significance of ayurveda lies in the way in which all the complex metabolic, physiological and pathological processes in the body have been explained by the normal or abnormal functioning of the three basic biological elements, vata, pitta and kapha. The practicality of this line of thinking is tremendous. It not only simplifies our understanding and approach to health and disease, but also makes it possible for the ayurvedic physician to practise and prescribe rationally on the basis of symptoms, even before disease becomes manifest. In other words, emphasis can be on prevention, rather than cure.

For example, if you complain of a burning sensation, the ayurvedic physician will apply cooling measures to subdue pitta. You will also be advised to avoid pungent, hot and sour foods and a hot environment. The practitioner of modern medicine, on the other hand, will tend to think of a B-complex deficiency and prescribe a vitamin B-complex supplement. If the burning *is* caused by a vitamin B deficiency, the results will be dramatic. If it is not, a modern doctor can often be at a loss as to what to prescribe. Similarly, when a child develops tetany (muscle spasms), it is interpreted as the result of a calcium deficiency by modern medicine and quickly corrected by giving injections of calcium. In ayurveda, the same tetany convulsions are interpreted as being due to increased vata, following decreasing kapha. The child would be treated by administering milk and ghee (clarified butter), which subdues vata and increases kapha, as well as increasing calcium. Although this treatment certainly takes time to build up calcium levels in the body, it also counters any magnesium or vitamin D deficiencies that may also exist and that give rise to the same symptoms as tetany. Calcium alone will not correct these deficiencies, whereas the administration of milk and ghee will.

Modern medicine and science have evolved from the gross to the minute, that is, from body organs to cells to molecules, and from molecules to energy. Ayurveda and the ancient philosophies of India have always looked at humankind and the universe as evolving from an unbroken wholeness, the universal soul which is also the precursor of universal energy. The three doshas theory is a reflection of this approach to understanding the truth.

left **EATING ON THE RUN IS ONE OF THE BAD HABITS OF MODERN LIFESTYLES THAT CAN CAUSE IMBALANCE IN YOUR DIGESTIVE CAPACITY. ALWAYS TAKE THE TIME TO SIT DOWN TO MEALS AND APPRECIATE AND SAVOUR WHAT YOU EAT**

The five subtypes of doshas

To simplify our understanding of the various roles the doshas play inside our body, each one has been conceived of as having five subtypes. Prana, udana, samana, vyana and apana are the five subtypes of vata. Pachaka, ranjaka, sadhaka, alochaka and bhrajaka are the five subtypes of pitta. Kledaka, avalambaka, bodhaka, tarpaka and shleshaka are the five subtypes of kapha. Here, the apana vata is said to be the controller of the other four types of vata. In the case of pitta, packaka pitta is the controller of the four other types of pitta. In kapha, avalambaka kapha is the most important of the subtypes.

Physical properties of the doshas

Doshas are also considered as substances with physical qualities and actions (karma), which are as follows:

Vata – dry, rough, cold, light, clear, transparent, not viscous, fine, penetrating

Pitta – hot, sharp, liquid (fluid), flowing, slightly oily, viscous, yellow and red

Kapha – oily, sticky, cold, heavy, coarse, stable, motionless, smooth and white

Five subtypes of vata

VATA SUBTYPE	LOCATION	NORMAL FUNCTIONS
Prana (Regulates cerebrospinal system)	Heart (special seat) Head, brain Lungs Ears, nose and tongue	Respiration Push food down the oesophagus Belching, sneezing, spitting
Udana (Regulates respiratory autonomics)	Larynx (special seat) Umbilical region Heart and lungs Throat	Sound, speech and singing Effort Affect the strength of the body
Samana (Regulates digestive autonomics)	Umbilical region (special seat) Stomach Intestines Channels carrying perspiration and urine, for example	Excite agni (digestive fire) Digest food Separate the products of digestion Send waste products downwards
Vyana (Regulates circulatory autonomics)	Throughout the body	Effects the circulation of blood and chyle (fluid composed of lymph and fat globules created during digestion) Effects movements of the body and the outflow of blood and perspiration from the body Yawning, blinking of the eyes
Apana (Regulates pelvic autonomics)	Rectum (special seat) Large intestine Bladder Organs of generation Thighs Umbilicus	Bear down the foetus Bring down urine, faeces, semen and menstrual blood Exert a downward pull upon the body's vayu (air)

Five subtypes of pitta

PITTA SUBTYPE	LOCATION	NORMAL FUNCTIONS
Pachaka	Duodenum	Digest food Reduce the food into lymph and excreta Supplement the other four pitta subtypes and thus maintain body heat
Ranjaka	Liver and spleen	Impart red colour to chyle (fluid containing lymph and emulsified fat) and convert it to blood
Sadhaka	Heart and brain	Help realize one's desires Maintain the intellect and memory
Alochaka	Eye	Maintain normal vision
Bhrajaka	Skin	Digest oily substances Irradiate the complexion

Five subtypes of kapha

KAPHA SUBTYPE	LOCATION	NORMAL FUNCTIONS
Kledaka	Stomach	Moisten food and break it down Gastric lubrication
Avalambaka	Thoracic cavity – heart and lungs	Protect the heart and lungs from excessive heat, thus enabling them to function properly Support the shoulderblades in their proper positions
Bodhaka	Root of the tongue Throat	Help in the perception of taste by keeping the tongue moist
Tarpaka	Skull and brain	Cool the different sense organs Cerebrospinal lubrication
Shleshaka	Joints	Keep the joints firmly united Lubricate and protect the different articulations

The influence of the three doshas

The table below summarizes the effects of the three
doshas on an individual's physical constitution (*prakruti*),
psychological constitution (*guna*), digestion, function
of the bowels and the six tastes.

DOSHA	PRAKRUTI (BODY TYPE)		THE THREE GUNAS (MENTAL TYPE)
	TYPE OF PRAKRUTI	MANIFESTATION	GUNA
VATA	Heena prakruti	Emaciated body and nervous nature	Satvic + rajas
PITTA	Madhyama prakruti	Overanxious nature	Satvic (in normalcy); rajas when aggravated
KAPHA	Uttama prakruti	Sound temperament	Satvic (in normalcy); tamas when aggravated
BALANCED DOSHAS	Sreshta prakruti	Best temperament	

DOSHA	DIGESTIVE CAPACITY		BOWEL FUNCTION	
	DIGESTIVE FIRE	TYPE OF DIGESTION	SANSKRIT TERM	ACTION ON BOWELS
VATA	Vishamagni	Variable	Krura kostha	Constipated bowels
PITTA	Teekshsnagni	Food digested too quickly	Mrudu kostha	Loose bowels
KAPHA	Mandagni	Unable to digest any food	Madhyama koshta	Normal bowel function
BALANCED DOSHAS	Samanagni	Normal digestion	Madhyama koshta	Normal bowel function

DOSHA	THE SIX TASTES	
	CONTROLLING TASTE	AGGRAVATING TASTE
VATA	Sweet, sour, salty	Pungent, bitter, astringent
PITTA	Astringent, bitter, sweet	Sour, salty, pungent
KAPHA	Pungent, bitter, astringent	Sweet, sour, salty

Your prakruti

Human life begins as a fertilized ovum. The sperm and ovum carry within them the constitution of both the parents. For example, at the time of conception, a sperm with vata dosha can inhibit some of the characteristics of an ovum of kapha dosha, that is, the dry, light, rough and mobile qualities of vata will suppress the unctuous, heavy, smooth and steady qualities of kapha. On the other hand, the cold quality, which is common to both doshas, would be aggravated, leading to extreme sensitivity to cold. The offspring in this case would inherit a vata-kapha constitution. If both father and mother, that is, sperm and ovum, were vata dominant, the progeny would inherit a dominant vata constitution. All the characteristics of vata would manifest in a far more aggravated form compared to those present in the parents.

Charaka, one of the founding fathers of ayurveda, observed the influence of genetic factors on the formation and overall development of the foetus. According to Charaka, your prakruti (body type or physical constitution) is fixed during the time of conception and remains unchanged throughout your life. The criteria of health vary with your prakruti. Also, if any parts of the chromosome or gene are not stable at conception or during pregnancy, the corresponding abnormalities of structure and functional disorders can be seen in the offspring.

How is your prakruti determined?

A combination of the five elements present during conception ultimately decides what your physical constitution is going to be. Other factors that influence the final outcome include the:

- Predominant dosha in sperm and ovum
- Time and season of conception
- Condition of the uterus
- Diet and behaviour of the expectant mother
- Lifestyle of the parents, their thoughts and even their occupations (which in turn influence the sperm and ovum)
- Racial type
- Country of origin and place of residence
- The age of the parents

Why is it important?

In ayurveda, your individual prakruti is considered very important, particularly in relation to disease. It determines the type of diseases to which you will be prone, how and in what manner those diseases will appear, any complications which may arise and your prognosis. Your prakruti also has an impact on how you respond to treatment.

These factors make it clear that determining and understanding your individual prakruti are crucial to receiving the correct ayurvedic diagnosis and treatment. It should always be a priority on the list of things to determine when you first visit an ayurvedic physician. Furthermore, no treatment should ever be prescribed without proper evaluation of your prakruti.

Classifications of prakruti

Four types of prakruti are recognized in ayurveda:

- Sama prakruti
- Vata prakrati
- Pitta prakruti
- Kapha prakruti

A perfect balance of the three doshas is said to be sama prakruti (balanced constitution). This is the ideal constitution, as the balanced state of each dosha neutralizes any negative or unwanted qualities, and supports and brings out the good qualities, so that the person leads a healthy life. If you have a sama prakruti, you will have the maximum immunity and ability to balance and deal with any physical or psychological change. Unfortunately, this desirable state of being is very rare.

What is generally seen in nature is a predominance of a particular dosha, leading to either vata prakruti, pitta prakruti or kapha prakruti. People with a predominance of any particular dosha are found to be more susceptible to diseases relating to those doshas. Hence vata people are susceptible to vata diseases, pitta people to pitta diseases and kapha people to kapha diseases.

Experience shows that the most common prakruti in an individual is that which involves the combination of two doshas. As a result, three more varieties of prakruti have been recognized. The constitutional types emerging from these combinations could be any of the following:

- vata-pitta type
- vata-kapha type
- kapha-pitta type

In ayurveda, these people are called *dwandaja* or *samsrasta prakruti* individuals. They exhibit combined physical, mental and emotional characteristics.

Features of each prakruti

The features of any prakruti are dependent on the qualities of the particular dosha to which it relates. Each quality has a specific effect on the formation of specific characteristics.

VATA PRAKRUTI

Vata is described as being dry, rough, light, mobile, abundant, swift, cold, coarse and non-shiny in quality. Therefore, people with a vata constitution would exhibit the following characteristics:

- Rough, dry skin
- Short body
- Lack of body strength
- Weak, low, hoarse voice
- Vigilance
- Lightness and unsteady movements
- Tall
- Small appetite
- Instability of joints, eyebrows, jaw, lips, tongue, head, shoulders, hands and feet. Movements of eyebrows, lips, hands and legs are exaggerated
- Intolerance to cold. People with a vata prakruti are often prone to cold hands and feet. It also produces stiffness in the body
- Coarse hair – usually short
- Small face, hands, feet, mouth and teeth
- Cracking in body joints
- Preference for sweet, sour, and salty tastes.
- Craving for warm food and warm drinks
- Liking for warm climates
- Irritability
- Dreams of running, jumping and climbing trees or mountains
- Inability to trust others readily
- Less control over their passions
- Unstable mind
- Weak sexual drive
- Prone to suffering from vata diseases

PITTA PRAKRUTI

Pitta is described as hot, sharp, liquid, fleshy, sour and pungent. People with a pitta constitution would exhibit the following characteristics:

- Intolerance to heat
- Facial skin is usually fair with moles, freckles, black patches, acne
- Excessive hunger and thirst
- Early appearance of wrinkles, grey hair and hair loss (alopecia)
- Soft, sparse and brown-coloured hair – usually short and scanty

- Heroism, valour and courage
- Prone to overeating and overimbibing
- Dislike of hard physical work
- Laxity and softness in joints and muscles
- Excess perspiration
- Bad breath and strong body odour
- Insufficient semen and inadequate sexual performance
- Preference for sweet, astringent and bitter tastes
- Craving for cold food and drinks and dislike of hot food and drinks
- Dislike of hot climates
- Dreams of gold, the sun, blazing fires, lightning, a glow in the sky, fights, quarrels and struggles
- Radiance, pride, irritability, argumentative, unbending, difficult to dominate and affectionate towards dependents
- Tendency towards impatience and aggression
- Moderate strength, wealth, life span, knowledge and understanding
- Prone to suffering from pitta diseases

KAPHA PRAKRUTI

Kapha is described as being unctuous, smooth, soft, sweet, solid, dull, rigid, heavy, cold, slimy and clear in quality. People with a kapha prakruti would exhibit the following characteristics:

- Oily, smooth, soft, delicate and fair skin
- Abundant seminal fluid
- Compact, sturdy build
- Good body strength and general immunity
- Slow speech and slow food intake
- Delayed initiation of action
- Heaviness and stability in movement
- Small appetite and thirst
- Lower body temperature and little perspiration
- Strong joints and ligaments
- Clear eyes and a clear voice
- Preference for pungent, bitter and astringent tastes
- Craving for dry and hot food
- Dislike of humid and cold climates
- Excellent memory, but slow comprehension
- Not easily excited
- Slow to form attachments to people or things, and vice versa
- Slow, sure walk with stable footing, comparable to the movement of a swan
- Large and attractive eyes
- Long, well-padded bones with large, robust joints
- Dreams of romantic events
- Prosperous, self-controlled, merciful, stable in friendship, lovable, generous, intelligent, strong and enthusiastic. Plenty of wealth, progeny and friends
- Prone to suffering from kapha diseases

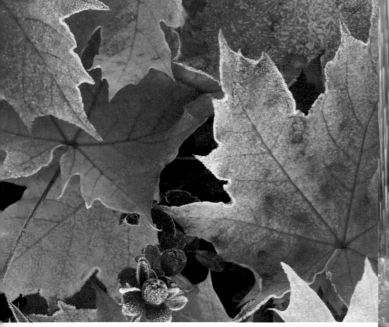

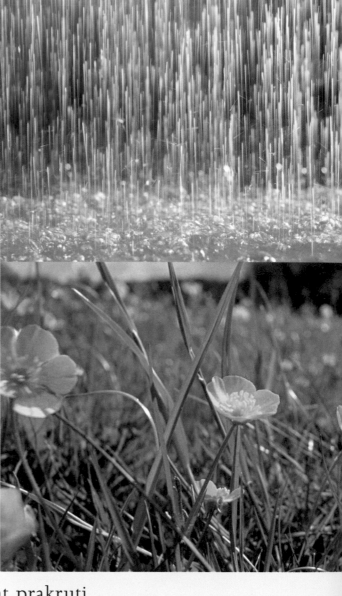

Prakruti and disease

One of the main benefits of identifying your prakruti (physical constitution) is that you can plan preventive approaches to specific dosha imbalances. After all, prevention is one of the key tenets of the ayurvedic system of healthcare. Also, as your prakruti involves features of both your body and mind, it is considered to be a vital part of ayurveda's holistic approach. Examples of some of the diseases particular to each prakruti are listed below.

Just as food, lifestyle and the time of day have profound effects on your prakruti and subsequently your health, so do the seasons. Vata people are more prone to illness during the rainy season, pitta people are more prone to illness during autumn and kapha people are more likely to be afflicted in spring.

Disorders associated with different prakruti

VATA PRAKRUTI
Ear ache
Arthritis of sacroiliac joint
Prolapsed rectum
Cracking of the soles
Colic pain
Stiffness of thighs
Hemiplegia (partial paralysis)
Sciatica
Sleeplessness
Unstable mentality

PITTA PRAKRUTI
Jaundice
Erysipelas
Haemorrhage
Skin inflammation
   of the feet
Urticaria
Stomatitis
Conjunctivitis
Pharyngitis
Fainting

KAPHA PRAKRUTI
Indigestion
Phlegm
Goitre
Obesity
Pallor
Excessive salivation
Excessive sleep
Arteriosclerosis (hardening
   of the arteries)
Loss of strength
Laziness

Prakruti and diet

As food has a profound influence on either increasing or decreasing a dosha, it is advisable to select food and drinks which help pacify the dosha imbalances of your particular prakruti. A list of some of the foods that should be favoured or avoided by each particular prakruti is given below. It is also important to consider good and bad food combinations (see page 78), and seasonal changes which may affect your prakruti.

Foods suitable for your prakruti

PRAKRUTI	FOODS TO FAVOUR	FOODS TO AVOID
VATA	Grains and pulses – rice, wheat, mung beans, red lentils Sugarcane, honey, jaggery Oils – sesame, corn, mustard, olive Dairy products – butter, ghee, cream Fruit – melons, bananas, oranges, pineapple, mango, papaya Vegetables – carrot, asparagus, cucumber, sweet potato, leafy greens Spices – black pepper, cinnamon, cumin, ginger (in small quantities) Meat, poultry and fish	Grains and pulses – corn, millet, oats Fruit – pears, dried fruits Vegetables – green peas, cabbage (in large quantities), cauliflower, potato, broccoli, aubergine (eggplant) Cold water Ice cream
PITTA	Grains and pulses – rice, wheat, barley, oats Oils – olive, sunflower, coconut Fruit – apples, grapes, cherries, avocado, oranges, mango Vegetables – artichokes, asparagus, broccoli, Brussels sprouts, cabbage, cucumber, okra (ladies' fingers), potato, pumpkin Spices – coriander, cinnamon (in small quantities), fenugreek Chicken, freshwater fish, turkey	Grains and pulses – corn, millet, brown rice Honey Oils – almond, sesame, corn, mustard Dairy products – yogurt, cheese, sour cream Fruit – papaya, peach, pineapple, melon, tomato Vegetables – onion, radish, spinach, garlic Spices – ginger, cumin
KAPHA	Grains and pulses – barley, corn, millet Honey Dairy products – low-fat milk Fruits – apple, pear, pomegranate Vegetables – beetroot, radish, aubergine (eggplant), bitter gourd, cucumber Spices – all spices, particularly hot ones such as black pepper or chilli Freshwater fish, chicken (white meat), turkey, rabbit, shrimp	Grains and pulses – wheat, rice (in large quantities) All oily items Fruit – melon, grapes, avocado, banana, tomato Vegetables – sweet potato Nuts

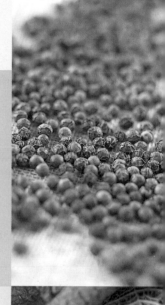

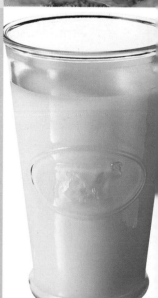

What is your prakruti?

It is best to have your individual prakruti assessed by a qualified ayurvedic practitioner. However, the following questions can act as a guide to determining your main dosha (or combination of doshas). The category which draws the most positive answers is your body type. If two of the categories are equally dominant, you are a combination of these doshas.

VATA TRAITS
- Do you perform activities very quickly?
- Are you bad at memorizing?
- Are you enthusiastic and vivacious by nature?
- Do you have a thin physique and not gain weight easily?
- Do you find it hard to make decisions?
- Do you tend to develop gas or become constipated easily?
- Are you prone to cold hands and feet?
- Are you frequently anxious or worried?
- Do you dislike cold weather?
- Are you intolerant of most people?
- Are you talkative and do you speak quickly?
- Does your mood change easily and are you somewhat emotional by nature?
- Do you often have difficulty in falling asleep or getting a sound night's sleep?
- Does your skin tends to be very dry, especially in the winter?
- Is your mind very active, sometimes restless, but also imaginative?
- Are your movements quick and active, and does your energy tend to come in bursts?
- Are you easily excitable?
- Left to your own devices, do your eating and sleeping habits tend to be irregular?
- Do you learn quickly, but also forget quickly?

PITTA TRAITS

- Do you consider yourself to be very efficient?
- Are you extremely precise and orderly in your activities?
- Are you strong-minded with a somewhat forceful manner?
- Are you of medium build and medium weight?
- Do you feel uncomfortable or easily fatigued in hot weather?
- Do you tend to perspire easily?
- Even though you might not always show it, do you become irritable or angry quite easily?
- If you skip a meal or a meal is delayed, do you become uncomfortable?
- Does one or more of the following describe your hair: greying or balding; thin, fine and straight; blond, reddish or sandy-coloured?
- Do you have a strong appetite?
- Do many people consider you stubborn?
- Are you very regular in your bowel habits? (It would be more common for you to have loose stools than to be constipated.)
- Do you become impatient very easily?
- Are you a perfectionist about details?
- Do you anger quite easily, but then quickly forget about it?
- Are you fond of cold foods, ice cream and ice-cold drinks?
- Are you more likely to feel that a room is too hot than too cold?
- Do you dislike foods that are very hot and spicy?
- Are you not as tolerant of disagreements as you should be?
- Do you enjoy challenges and show great determination?
- Do you tend to be quite critical of others and also of yourself?

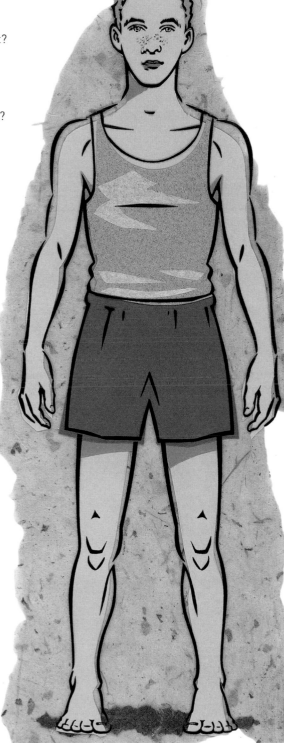

KAPHA TRAITS

- Is your natural tendency to do things in a slow and relaxed fashion?
- Do you gain weight more easily than most people and lose it more slowly?
- Do you have a placid and calm disposition – you are not easily ruffled and not easily angered?
- Can you skip meals easily without any significant discomfort?
- Do you have a tendency towards excess mucus, phlegm, chronic congestion, asthma or sinus problems?
- Do you need at least eight hours sleep in order to function comfortably the next day?
- Do you sleep very deeply?
- Are you slower to learn than some people, but with excellent retention and a long memory?
- Do you have a tendency towards being plump?
- Does cool, damp weather bother you?
- Is your hair thick, dark and wavy?
- Is your body large and solidly built?
- Do the following words described you well: serene, sweet-natured, affectionate and forgiving?
- Do you have a slow digestion, which makes you feel heavy after eating?
- Do you have very good stamina and a steady level of energy?
- Do you generally walk with a slow, measured gait?
- Do you have a tendency towards oversleeping and grogginess upon waking, and are you generally slow to get going in the morning?
- Are you a slow eater and slow and methodical in your actions?

The three gunas

When discussing your constitution as an individual, it is essential also to take into consideration your mental or psychological constitution. While the three doshas are integral to the nature of your physical constitution, the basis of your mental constitution, or manasa prakruti, are the three gunas of the mind – satvic, rajas and tamas. In ayurveda, they are invariably known as *satwas*. Broadly, they are classified into three types:

- Satvic satwa – noble and strong
- Rajasic satwa – human and egotistical
- Tamasic satwa – human and vulnerable

Every individual has aspects of each of these satwas, but it is the most dominant one that forms our individual psychological constitution.

Unlike your prakruti, or physical constitution, your psychological constitution is not strictly genetic – although the circumstances of you conception can sometimes have an influence. However, through religious and spiritual practice, you can overcome any temperamental constraints and become *trigunateet* or *purushottam*, that is, an ideal person endowed with godly qualities and character.

Learning to keep your three satwas – satvic, rajas and tamas – in harmony will lead to a the healthiest state of mind. If they are out of equilibrium, various mental disorders and disease can follow. Mental disturbance is caused by an imbalance of the rajas and tamas satwas. As satvic is believed to be the pure or highest state of mind, it cannot be considered out of balance or in excess. Of course, everyone should aspire to being fully satvic, but this is very rare in practice. Nonetheless, the practise of living mindfully and ethically, meditating and being aware and responsible for your actions, all bring you nearer to this ideal state of mind.

In ayurveda, striving for a balanced mental state is equally important to looking after your physical wellbeing. After all, mind and body are inextricably linked when it comes to health and happiness. Purity of mind, body and spirit is sought through diet and lifestyle, detoxification, yoga and meditation.

Characteristics of satvic satwa

This guna is characterized by consciousness, clarity, pleasure and lightness. It is linked to the perception of knowledge and is free from disease. Satvic people are positive, respectful and filled with an inner peace. Other characteristics of satvic satwa are:

- Steady and pure mind
- Religious nature
- Righteousness
- Good manners and good characteristics
- Great degree of self-control
- Not easily upset or angered
- Respect for teachers, elders and parents
- Clear intellect
- Follows the path of truth
- Pursues knowledge, proficiency and skill
- Takes correct decisions after careful and mature thinking
- Super-ego dominates over id and ego

Characteristics of rajasic satwa

Motion and stimulation characterize rajas. Desires, ambitions and fickleness are the result of this guna. Psychiatric illness can result from an imbalance in rajas. Other characteristics of rajasic satwa are:

- Egotistical, proud and ambitious
- Tendency to rule others
- Hardworking, but lacking proper planning and direction
- Calm and patient only as long as their interests are not affected
- Friendly and faithful only to those who are helpful to them
- Emotions such as anger, joy, attachment and jealousy dominate
- Suffer frequent emotional outbursts, so that mental energy is wasted and fatigue sets in
- Ego usually dominates over id and super-ego

Characteristics of tamasic satwa

Heaviness and resistance are the main features of tamasic satwa. Excess tamas can cloud perception and the mind's activities. Other characteristics are:

- Less intelligent
- Depressed frame of mind
- Prone to laziness and apathy
- Tendency to feel sleepy, even during the daytime
- Extremely greedy and irritable
- No consideration for others
- May harm others to safeguard their own interests
- Follows the path of least resistance and given to eating and drinking too much, oversleeping and having sex to excess
- Id dominates over ego and super-ego

Understanding the six tastes

There are six tastes according to ayurveda. Taste is a specific quality of the basic element of water and can only be perceived by the tongue (taste buds). In ayurveda, each taste is a combination of two basic elements. This means that understanding the six tastes is another way of acquiring knowledge about the five elements – air, space, fire, water and earth.

The six tastes and their elemental combinations are:

- Sweet (*madhura*) – earth and water
- Sour (*amla*) – earth and fire
- Salty (*lavana*) – water and fire
- Pungent (*katu*) – air and fire
- Bitter (*tikta*) – air and space
- Astringent (*kashaya*) – air and earth

The six tastes act on the body in different ways: through their properties or qualities, through changes which take place during or after digestion, or through their potency, and so on. For example, the sweet taste, with its dominant elements of earth and water, is a builder of those tissues which are formed from earth and water. Sweet-tasting substances strengthen kapha dosha (made from earth and water), but weaken pitta and vata.

The properties of taste

- Sweet taste contributes to longevity and increases the quality of kapha in the body. It is endowed with the attributes that particularly pertain to the material principles of earth and water.
- Sour taste increases the taste of food and salivation processes. Its attributes belong to the principles of earth and fire.
- Salty taste imparts a greater relish for food and is possessed of corrective virtues. It is mostly endowed with the attributes that characterize the elementary principles of water and fire.
- Pungent taste destroys obesity and intestinal parasites, is antitoxic in its character and is a good curative for skin diseases. It strongly possesses attributes that belong to the principles of air and fire. It acts as a sedative and lessens the quantity of fat, milk and semen.
- Bitter taste is a good appetite stimulant and also a good purifying agent in respect of ulcers. It has the virtue of drying up pus, mucus and fat, for example. The specific attributes of air and space predominate the bitter taste.

- Astringent taste lessens secretions from the mucus membrane. The properties of earth and air are dominant in it.

THE TEN PAIRS OF QUALITIES

There are 20 fundamental qualities, organized into ten pairs of opposites, which are used in ayurvedic analysis. The pairs are: heaviness/lightness, coldness/hotness, unctuousness/roughness, dullness/sharpness, stability/mobility, softness/hardness, smoothness/coarseness, non-sliminess/sliminess, minuteness/grossness and solidity/liquidity. The qualities in a pair each exert an influence upon the other.

The properties of the six tastes corresponding to the 20 qualities are listed below:

- Sweet – heavy + hot + oily + gelatinous
- Sour – heavy + hot + oily
- Salty – heavy + hot + oily + sharp
- Pungent – light + hot + dry
- Bitter – light + cold + dry + subtle + fine
- Astringent – light + cold + dry

The action of the tastes in ayurveda

Ayurveda explains the relationship of tastes to the doshas as a set of three tastes which can increase or decrease a particular dosha.

VATA

The three tastes containing the basic element of air – pungent, astringent and bitter – strengthen and increase vata and all activities relating to the cleansing of the body channels, penetration and movement. The tastes that do not contain the basic element of air – sweet, sour and salty – weaken and sedate vata, while at the same time building up kapha.

PITTA

The three tastes containing the basic element of fire – sour, salty and pungent – strengthen pitta and the functions associated with it, such as a rise in body temperature, all metabolic processes (digestion of food) and the cleansing of the body channels. The tastes that do not contain the basic element of fire – bitter, sweet or astringent – weaken and decrease pitta.

KAPHA

The three tastes, sweet, sour and salty, increase the action of kapha, because they all contain one or both of the basic elements of earth and water (like kapha itself). The bitter and pungent tastes sedate and decrease kapha while increasing vata, because they both contain the elements of air and space.

Whatever strengthens vata will weaken kapha, and vice versa. Even though the astringent taste has the specific elemental configuration of air and earth, it is considered in the group together with bitter and pungent, because the air element is the most dominant of the two.

The action of tastes on *agni* (digestive fire), body tissues, body channels and waste products are listed on pages 38–9, together with their positive and negative actions. The negative action of taste can only be seen when the particular taste is experienced excessively or continuously over a very long period.

Understanding the concept of the six tastes is critical, as it is the basis of all pharmacological and dietary principles. Ayurvedic medicines, herbal remedies and dietary substances are based solely on knowledge of the six tastes and its related factors, such as their qualities or physical properties, potency, post-digestive effect and specific action. The predominant tastes of some drugs and foodstuffs are given below.

Drugs and foodstuffs with predominant tastes

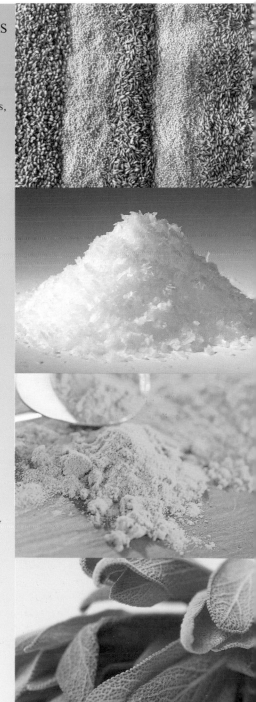

TASTE	DRUG OR FOODSTUFF
SWEET	Barley, butter, coconut, cream, dates, grapes, ghee (clarified butter), lentils, marshmallow plant, maize, milk, millet, oats, sesame oil, rice, rye, shatavari (*Asparagus racemosus* Willd.), sugarcane, wheat
SOUR	Cheese, citrus fruits, Indian gooseberry (*amalaki*), lemon, lime, morello cherries, pickles, pomegranate, raspberry, sea blackthorn, sorrel, tomato, turmeric, vinegars, yogurt
SALTY	Rock salt, sea salt, table salt
PUNGENT	Asafoetida (*hing*), black pepper, black mustard, caraway, cayenne, camomile, chilli, cinnamon, cumin, dill, garlic, ginger, holy (Thai) basil, horseradish, Indian lemongrass, long pepper (*pippali*), nutmeg, onion, paprika, radish
BITTER	Aconitum, aloe, bitter gourd (*karela*), brahmi (*gotukola* or Indian pennywort), Brussels sprouts, coriander, fenugreek, gentian, goldenseal, neem, rhubarb, spinach and other leafy green vegetables, Swiss chard, turmeric, valerian, vetiver
ASTRINGENT	Apples, asparagus, aubergine (eggplant), bilwa (*Aegle marmelos* Corr.), broccoli, celery, fennel, gum of myrrh, haritaki (*Terminalia chebula*), honey, leek, oak, sage, walnut, St John's wort, whortleberries, witch hazel

TASTE	ACTION OF TASTE ON DOSHAS (bioregulating principles)	ACTION OF TASTE ON DIGESTIVE FIRE	ACTION OF TASTE ON BODY TISSUES
SWEET Pleasant, strengthening, soothes the mouth	Increases kapha; reduces vata and pitta	Because of its heavy nature, its effect on the digestive fire is to slow the digestion process. Its oily, gelatinous nature gives it a blocking effect (like constipation) on the ducts	The only taste that stimulates anabolic activity in the body by increasing all the tissues and vitality in general
SOUR Causes salivation, perspiration and a burning sensation in the mouth and throat. It cleanses the mouth and stimulates the appetite	Stimulates pitta and kapha; reduces vata	Strengthens agni, the biological fire, and therefore aids digestion	Stimulates activities of agni and has a decreasing effect on semen. It is not recommended as a tonic
SALTY Retains water, softens and is easily soluble. It stimulates the appetite and produces a burning sensation in the mouth and throat	Stimulates pitta and kapha; reduces vata	Increases the digestive power of agni and improves the appetite	Has a catabolic effect and acts by increasing water content. It causes a physical sensation of laxness in the body and assists in breaking down the body tissue
PUNGENT Causes salivation, headache and a tingling sensation in the tongue	Strengthens vata and pitta; reduces kapha	Strengthens the digestive fire and therefore sharpens the appetite and promotes digestion	Catabolic, drying and absorptive
BITTER Stimulates the appetite and cleanses the mouth. It also produces dryness in the mouth and overshadows all other tastes	Reinforces vata; reduces pitta and kapha	Acts on the digestive fire and supports the vata located in the stomach and intestine by absorbing the mucus-producing kapha	The action on the tissue is catabolic. It depletes fat, plasma, tissue, bone marrow and reproductive tissues
ASTRINGENT Produces stiffness and traction in the tongue and throat, dryness in the mouth, pain in the cardiac region and heaviness	Reinforces vata; reduces pitta through cold and kapha through dryness	It has no adverse effect on the digestive fire	Helps in the healing process. It decreases the volume of urine because of its absorption properties, and helps heal wounds on the skin

ACTION OF TASTE ON WASTE PRODUCTS		ACTION OF TASTE ON THE BODY CHANNEL	POSITIVE AND NEGATIVE ACTIONS OF TASTES	
PREDOMINANT ELEMENT	ACTION		POSITIVE EFFECTS	DISORDERS CAUSED BY EXCESSIVE USE - NEGATIVE EFFECTS
Earth	Laxative	If the digestion is normal, the sweet taste acts as a tonic and the channels of the body remain open. The sweet taste can have the effect of obstructing the channels under some conditions. When this happens, bitter and pungent substances are taken to cleanse the ducts and regulate digestion	Promotes weight increase; imparts vitality; body tonic; laxative; diuretic; healing; brain tonic	Obesity; anorexia; respiratory disorders; goitre; swelling of lymph nodes; diabetes; intestinal worms and filaria
Earth	Diuretic	No specific effect on the channels; instead, it may contribute to obstructing them	Stimulates appetite; expels wind (carminative); combats anorexia; promotes bleeding (anticoagulant)	Blood disorders; swelling; inflammations; burning sensation; skin diseases; anaemia; haemorrhage; vertigo; vision defects
Earth	Carminative (relieves flatulence)	Cleanses the body channels. This taste has no absorbing property, but liquifies the solid mass and helps to expel it because of its sharp quality	Moistening; stimulates appetite; digestive; expectorant; harmful to semen; diuretic; contaminates blood	Impotence; greying hair; falling hair; haemorrhage; skin diseases; erysipelas; gastric disorders
Air	Constipating	Has a cleansing effect on the body channels. This is due to its air and fire elements, which absorb the fluid and expel the obstructive material and are responsible for gentle expectoration (coughing up)	Cleanses mouth; stimulates appetite; digestive; promotes weight loss; destroys or expels intestinal worms; nerve stimulant; useful in dyspepsia; cardiac and skin disorders	Impotence; vertigo; unconsciousness; debility; thirst; burning sensation; mental weakness
Air	Antidiuretic	Cleanses the body channels and ducts. It acts in the same manner as the pungent taste by absorbing the fluid and slimy material due to vata because of its inherent dry quality. Its space element creates space and its power of penetration gives it access to the smallest channels	Stimulates appetite; digestive; reduces fever; destroys or expels intestinal worms; removes pus, toxins and serious discharges; useful in anorexia, skin diseases and easing burning sensation	Emaciation; debility; vertigo; dryness of the mouth; neurological diseases; mental weakness; nausea
Air	Causes obstruction in passing gas	No particular effect on the channels; instead, it may participate in obstructing the channels and pores	Astringent; absorbent; healing; harmful to semen; antidiuretic; normalizes skin pigmentation	Dryness of mouth; cardiac pain; impotence; neurological disorders; obstruction of channels (for example, constipation)

Causes of disease in ayurveda

Good health is an ideal state to which we all aspire. Unfortunately however, illness and disease are an ever present reality for many people. Knowingly or unknowingly, we all fall prey to illness or disease at some time in our lives. Often, it can seem that with each illness, our bodies manage to develop some resistance and immunity towards it. In fact, in this sense, becoming sick is the body's way of knowing how to be well and fit.

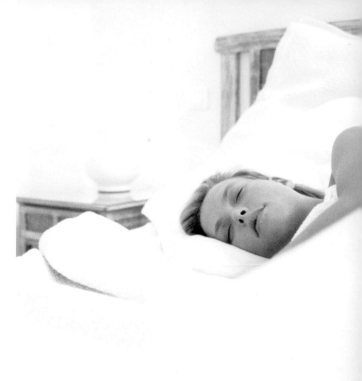

Disharmony of the body elements causes disease. The body elements to be considered here are the doshas, tissues (*dhatus*), waste products (*malas*), digestive fire (*agni*) and channels (*srotas*). There are certain quantitative, qualitative and functional norms for these elements in the body. When they decrease or increase in comparison to their normal values, disease sets in. When the body's psychological components stop functioning normally, disease also sets in, as a result of the inextricable link between body and mind.

Vata, pitta and kapha are the doshas relating to our physical bodies or physical constitution (prakruti). When the doshas are out of balance or in an abnormal state, they cause physical disease (see page 30). Satvic, rajas and tamas are the mental gunas relating to our psychological or mental constitution (see page 35). When either rajas or tamas is out of equilibrium, or in an abnormal state, this can cause psychological or mental illness, or lead to physical disease as a result of the mind's disharmony and the knock-on effect this has on our physical health.

The ayurvedic texts give detailed descriptions of the causes of imbalance or abnormality of the doshas and the signs and symptoms that appear when they are destabilized, that is, increased or decreased (see pages 43–5). Apart from these specific causes of dosha imbalance or abnormality, ayurveda also specifies three general causes for any disease. They are:

- Indiscriminate use of senses and their objects
- Seasonal variations, cosmic effects and time
- Error of intellect, inability to discriminate between wholesome and unwholesome thoughts and actions, and indulging in diets and behaviour conducive to the development of disease

Of these three, the error of intellect (*prajnaparadha*) is considered to be the foremost cause of any disease.

What is prajnaparadha?

In ayurvedic terminology, *prajnaparadha* is the failure to coordinate *dhi*, *dhriti* and *smriti*. *Dhi* is the power of discrimination between right and wrong, good and bad, useful and harmful. *Dhriti* is the ability to retain the experience in memory. *Smriti* is memory or experiences. The three combined contribute to the reflection, registration and recall ability of our psychic system and experience. Experience adds to knowledge, which is built upon during consciousness. In any given situation, it is this experience or knowledge which guides the action (karma) of an individual. In strict medical parlance, mind controls physiology.

If, for any reason, any one or indeed a combination of these powers becomes inert or blunt, the messages released from our consciousness are not passed on to the mind. In this situation, intuition is replaced by instinct. The consequence is that the individual indiscriminately indulges in unwholesome foods and practices, which in turn invites disease.

The reasons for poor judgement and the inability to recall past experience and learn from mistakes have been expressed very clearly in the ancient Indian philosophical and religious text the *Bhagavad Gita*: 'When man constantly thinks of sense objects and the pleasure derived from it he develops attachment to them. This causes 'possessiveness', which in turn creates anger. This hostility leads to loss of judgement, which causes loss of memory. Man perishes because of memory loss.'

Body and mind are closely interlinked. The three doshas (vata, pitta and kapha) bear psychological as well as physical expressions or functions. Vata's psychological expression is enthusiasm, pitta's are lustre, cheerfulness and intellect, while Kapha's psychological expressions are forgiveness, memory based on experience, the intelligence to discriminate and non-acquisitiveness.

The seeds of all disease are sown in the mind. Every disease creates a mental transformation before it manifests as a physical imbalance. The psychological functions of the doshas are initially disturbed. First, non-acquisitiveness – one of kapha's psychological expressions – is lost or reversed. As a result, greed sets in, leading to overindulgence of the things which stimulate our senses, food and the accumulation of wealth, followed by fear and the worry of protecting and retaining it. Thus greed precedes attachment, which is developed by constantly thinking about sense objects. Although we are all advised to lead a life of 'resignation', your mind becomes focussed on sensual pleasures and creates attachment.

Attachment leads to accumulation and possessiveness due to the failure of kapha to retain the experience in memory. This follows the failure of another of kapha's psychological expressions, forgiveness. When any hindrance arises during the process of accumulation and hoarding, anger automatically develops and, as a result, the ability to forgive – the virtue of the fearless person – will be lost. Material greed makes people fearful and so they lose the quality of *kshama* (patience and tolerance). Excessive anger leads to loss of judgement and loss of happiness. All these end in a loss of enthusiasm, from where the physical cycle of disease starts. These are the initial and discrete psychological imbalances that precede the onset of the development of any disease. In ayurveda, the concept of *prajnaparadha* is used to explain the cause of the onset of any disease.

The development of disease

According to ayurveda, the body is an expression of consciousness. This consciousness creates the desire for survival, which is biologically fulfilled by ingestion, digestion and assimilation of food. This is where agni (digestive fire, or metabolism) plays its role. In the development, or pathogenesis, of any disease, agni is first impaired, either due to overeating or to worry, sorrow, fear or anger. Impaired agni causes indigestion, which, in turn, causes improperly formed chyle (fluid composed of lymph and emulsified fat globules created during digestion), leading to functional obstruction in the body's channels. In this way, metabolic disturbances lead to diseases of the body's organs and its channels.

In ayurvedic parlance, pathogenesis is called *samprapti*. The process has six stages: accumulation, provocation, circulation, localization, manifestation and complications. The doshas accumulate in their specific places according to the different causes of their increase. The *ama* (toxins or metabolic waste), formed by improperly functioning agni, joins the accumulated doshas. These doshas undergo certain fermentative changes, through which they overflow and begin spreading, or circulating, within the body. Wherever these circulating doshas find weaker sites or channels, they begin to localize. This process is known as *sthana samsraya*. It is at this stage that the unbalanced dosha and susceptible tissue join hand in hand to cause the early symptoms of a disease. The functions of any channels that are related to the susceptible tissue also show abnormal functioning, whether it be too much, too little or no function at all. This adds to the manifestation of a disease, with its full-blown signs and symptoms. During each of these stages, if your body's signals are properly observed and sufficient precautions are taken in terms of food, rest and lifestyle, your body will heal itself and nullify the dosha imbalances. If not, complications may develop, ultimately leading to death if left untreated.

In short, disease is an imbalance. Any decrease or increase of the normal state of the doshas is disease. When there is an increase, symptoms of that increase will naturally also be increased. A decreased dosha, on the other hand, loses its normal functions. The increase or decrease can be quantitative, qualitative, organic or functional. Ayurvedic treatment aims to boost decreased doshas and subdue increased ones, so as to restore and maintain balance, normality, harmony and equilibrium – in other words, health.

Importantly, ayurveda attaches equal significance to the physical and psychological components of the body. As ignorance breeds greed, great emphasis is placed on it as a primary cause of all disease. This does not mean that ayurvedic principles do not also acknowledge that micro-organisms, injury or trauma, and poisons can cause disease. Even the iatrogenic nature of disease (that is, illness caused by the actions of a doctor) was recognized in the ancient texts.

Pathways or tracts of diseases

According to the principles of ayurveda, the origin and manifestation of disease depend upon five things:

- Causative factors
- The doshas
- Condition and susceptibility of tissues and waste products of digestion and metabolism
- Potency and condition of various channels
- Pathways or tracts of disease

The pathways, or *rogamargas* as they are known in ayurveda, are a unique and important consideration in the ayurvedic system. There are three pathways of disease known as:

- Interior tract
- Exterior tract
- Middle tract

The prognosis and instability of a disease, as well as specific treatment interventions, are mainly dependent on these pathways. Disease in the interior tract is said to be at the disease origin site – the treatment approach in this case is quite straightforward. The other two pathways are the sites of manifestation of diseases, considered to be more deep-seated in the body. When a disease is in the exterior or middle tract, ayurvedica herbal medicine alone is not enough. Special approaches such as purification or detoxification are also needed.

Classification of diseases

The ancient ayurvedic texts have classified disease according to the cause, nature, effect, treatment and so on. The classification described in the *Sushruta Samhita* is considered to be the most comprehensive.

In ayurveda, disease is equated to misery, which is another indication of ayurveda's recognition of the complex link between mind and body. In other words, health relates to happiness and disease relates to unhappiness. This theory is interlinked with the theory of good conduct, or karma. According to Sushruta, there are three kinds of misery a person experiences as a result of his or her actions:

- Adhyatmika – pertaining to present body and life
- Adibhoutika – caused by external elements
- Adidaniska – caused by a previous life

These three categories of misery give rise to seven groups of disease:

- Genetic disorders – for example, asthma, epilepsy, some mental illnesses, haemophilia
- Congenital diseases – such as congenital deafness and blindness
- Constitutional diseases – diseases brought about by the actions of the three doshas or by one of the mental gunas of rajas and tamas
- Traumatic – disorders caused by external injury or due to poisons or germs
- Seasonal disorders – for example, sunstroke, frostbite, rheumatic diseases
- Natural disorders – including senility, osteoarthritis
- Infectious and spiritual disorders – such as epidemic diseases and sexually transmitted diseases

In most ayurvedic texts, diseases are classified as:

- Vata type
- Pitta type
- Kapha type
- Diseases due to a combination of two doshas
- Tridosha-type diseases (where all three doshas are unbalanced)
- Rakta type (due to contamination of the blood)

Diseases arising due to an imbalance of an individual dosha are known as *nana* diseases. There are 80 vata diseases, 40 pitta diseases and 20 kapha diseases. Most diseases fall under the first three classifications of a specific dosha type, or perhaps a combination.

The study of disease in ayurveda

Ayurveda has adopted a systemic and methodical way of understanding disease. This includes:

- Aetiology or the causes of disease
- Prodromal (early) symptoms
- Symptomatology
- Aggravating and alleviating factors/therapeutic test
- Pathogenesis or development of a disease
- Prognosis
- Complications
- Sequaelae (any disease or abnormality arising as a result of a pre-existing disease)
- Management
- Prevention

Disease is a gradual process and not a sudden event. The nature of onset, site of origin and manifestations, disease pathways and nomenclature are crucial – all are systematically presented and dealt with in ayurveda. A skilled ayurvedic physician is often able to recognize and treat disease before it becomes manifest.

Clinical manifestation of unbalanced doshas

DECREASED VATA

Desire for rough, light, pungent, bitter and/or astringent food
Exhaustion
Laziness
Drowsiness
Diminished sensation
Sluggish movements
Weakness in digestive power
Symptoms of relative increase of kapha dosha

AGGRAVATED VATA

Desire for hot things
Weakness
Darkening of the skin
Loss of weight
Loss of strength
Rough voice
Hoarse voice
Constipation
Distension of the abdomen
Paralysis
Insomnia
Tremors
Twitching
Carrying out irrelevant task
Giddiness
Defective motor functions
Defective sensory functions

EXCESSIVELY INCREASED VATA

Feeling of exhaustion
Excessive thirst
Goose skin
Roughness
Astringent taste in the mouth
Reddish discoloration
Blackish discoloration
Cavity formation
Prolapse of different organs
Dilation of organs
Retention of secretions
Retention of waste products
Loss of sensation
Pain – pricking, colicky, acute
Contraction
Tremors

DECREASED PITTA

Loss of appetite
Coldness of body
Hypoacidity – hypochlorhydria, achlorhydria
Hypothermia
Loss of lustre

AGGRAVATED PITTA

Generalized weakness
Desire for cold things
Jaundice (yellowish discoloration of skin, nails, urine, stools)
Insomnia
Unconsciousness
Increased (voracious) appetite
Burning sensation
Hyperthermia
Decay

EXCESSIVELY INCREASED PITTA

Feeling of exhaustion
Increased heat
Redness
Wetness
Burning sensation
Excessive sweating
Excessive discharges
Suppuration (discharge of pus from a wound or sore)
Sour taste in the mouth
Discoloration – yellowish, bluish, greenish
Delirium
Unconsciousness

DECREASED KAPHA

Increased roughness
Desire for sweet things
Craving for oily foods
Excessive thirst
Feeling of emptiness
Cardiomegaly (abnormal increase in the size of the heart)
Weakness of the joints
Giddiness
General weakness
Insomnia
Dislocation of the joints

AGGRAVATED KAPHA

Diseases of the respiratory system – coughing, breathlessness
Pallor
Cold skin
Excessive salivation
Weak digestive power
Affection of the joints
Laziness
Drowsiness

EXCESSIVELY INCREASED KAPHA

Hardness
Coldness
Viscousness
Heaviness
Sensation of tightening
Sensation as if thick paste is applied
Itching
Oedema (swelling)
Whitish discoloration
Sweet taste in the mouth
Salty taste in the mouth
Chronic disease
Excessive sleep
Numbness
Rigidity

Causes of increased dosha

There are a number of causes which can increase each of the doshas. Environmental factors such as the season and the time of day play their part, as does your age. While these things are a part of the natural rhythms of life and in a sense are unchanging, it is still important to be aware of their influence. There are other causative factors, such as the food we eat and the lifestyle we lead, over which we do have more control. These can be harnessed to increase dosha for a positive impact when necessary, or they can be reduced or avoided entirely if the increase in the respective dosha has a negative impact.

	VATA	PITTA	KAPHA
Environment	Cold, dry breeze, storms, cloudy weather	Heat, dust, smoke, dry climate	Rain, cold and humidity
Season	Summer and rainy seasons	Summer, autumn and rainy seasons	Spring and winter
Time of day	Afternoon – 2 pm to 6 pm	Midday – 10 am to 2 pm	Morning – 6 am to 10 am
Time of night	Late night – 2 am to 6 am	Midnight – 10 pm to 2 am	Early evening – 6 pm to 10 pm
Relation to meals	After food is completely digested	During digestion	Immediately after meals
Diet Seeds and pulses	Most dried beans, except red lentils	Toor dal, urid dal	Sesame seeds, urid dal
Cereals	Barley, buckwheat, corn, millet, rye	Buckwheat, brown rice, corn, millet	Pasta, rice (brown and white), wheat
Vegetables	Artichoke, aubergine (eggplant), Brussels sprouts, broccoli, cabbage, cauliflower, leafy greens, onion, radish, sweet peppers, turnip	Beet greens, beets (raw), chillies, garlic, mustard greens, radish, spinach (uncooked), sweetcorn, turnip	Courgettes (zucchini), cucumber, sweet potato, pumpkin
Fruits	Apples (uncooked), dried fruit, pears, watermelon	Sour fruits in general, lemons, oranges, tamarind	Avocado, dates, coconut
Fats and oils	Flaxseed	Corn, safflower, sesame	Ghee (clarified butter), olive
Meat		Beef, lamb, pork, saltwater fish	Beef, lamb, pork, saltwater fish, seafood in general
Milk and dairy products		Buttermilk, cheese (hard), whey, yogurt	Butter, cheese, ghee (clarified butter), ice cream, milk, soured cream, yogurt

	VATA	PITTA	KAPHA
Alcohol and wines	Some types of wines		Most wines and alcohol
Miscellaneous	Caraway, insufficient or dry food, white sugar	Black pepper, jaggery (palm sugar), molasses	Jaggery (palm sugar), maple syrup, molasses, sugar
General diet-related principles	Light diet, fasting, irregular diet, inadequate diet	Fasting, penance, incompatible diet, indigestion, burnt food	Indulging in spicy food, drinking excessive amounts of water in general and at night, eating too much of a nourishing diet, indigestion
Panchakarma	Following excessive use of panchakarma		
Natural urges	Suppression or induction of natural urges		
Psychological factors	Fear, sorrow, eagerness, anger, worry, study, trouble, excessive joy	Anger, fear, sorrow, envy	Laziness, excessive joy
Qualities Taste	Astringent, bitter, pungent	Sour, salty, pungent	Sweet, sour, salty
Veerya	Cold	Hot	Cold
Qualities	Dry, light, clean and constipating food	Hot, light and fermenting food	Semi-solid, oily, heavy, moist, soft, bulky, smooth and slimy food
Physical action Activity	Excessive physical activity	Excessive physical activity	Little physical activity
Exercise	Excessive exercise, plus: injury, swimming, carrying heavy loads, travelling, adventure sports	Excessive exercise, plus: exposure to the sun	No exercise, lack of exercise, laziness, rest in excess
Speech	Loud and excessive	Excessive	Little
Sex	Excessive	Excessive	Little
Sleep	Lack of sleep, lying awake at night	Lack of sleep	Excessive sleeping during the day, as well as at night
Age	Old age	Youth	Childhood

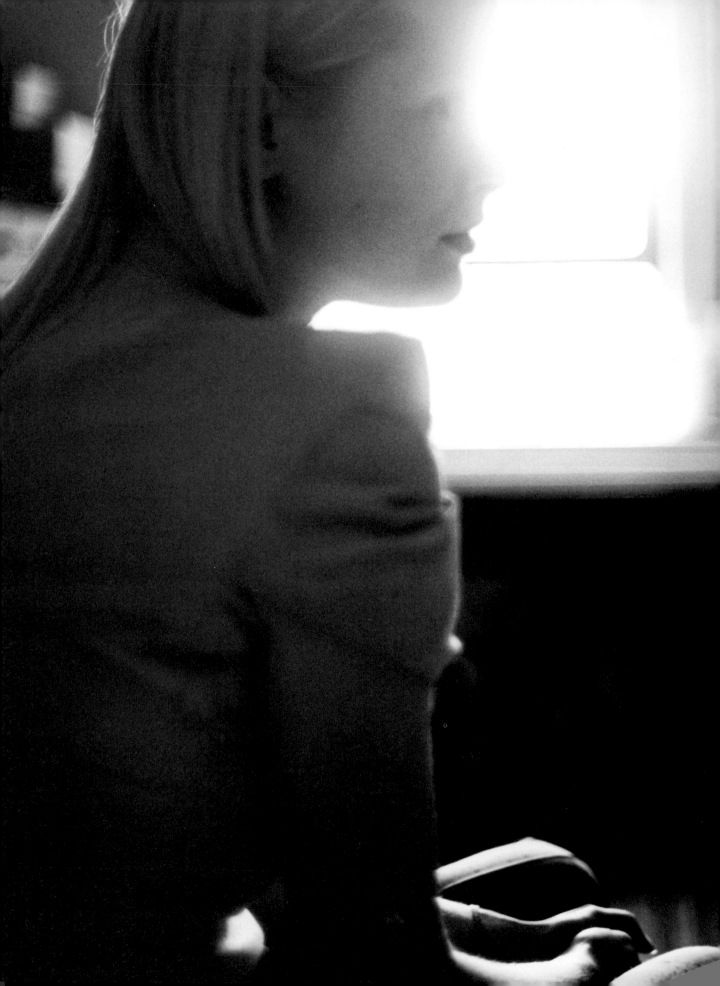

3 ayurvedic consultations and diagnosis

In ayurvedic medicine, diagnosis of illness is based on the practitioner directly observing the body and personality of a patient. Traditionally, a student of ayurveda must live and study with a fully qualified teacher in order to absorb completely the knowledge necessary for this most ancient art. While diagnosis is definitely an art in terms of the more subtle information that can be acquired, it still needs to be structured scientifically, using specific expertise and skills that can be developed.

Ayurvedic diagnosis is primarily concerned with the understanding of the three doshas. All the diagnostic methods review either the harmony or disharmony of the doshas in terms of excess or depletion. Each person is seen as an individual, not as an average statistic. Your individual constitution and your mental traits form your unique psychosomatic being, an important factor recognized in ayurvedic medicine before any attempt at diagnosis is made.

The ayurvedic consultation is a process aimed at individual health assessment and diagnosis. It involves the ayurvedic practitioner taking your medical history and performing a thorough clinical examination. You will be interviewed in a serene, quiet and peaceful consultation room. This is very important, as it helps to develop a better doctor–patient relationship, which is key not only to successful treatment, but also to your long-term commitment to the principles and practices of ayurveda. You need to be completely comfortable with, and have confidence in, your ayurvedic practitioner – this is vital to them eliciting the relevant and often very personal information necessary for diagnosis and treatment.

left **THE PATIENT MUST FEEL TOTAL CONFIDENCE IN THE DOCTOR, SO THAT AN ACCURATE DIAGNOSIS CAN BE MADE AND THE CORRECT COURSE OF TREATMENT CAN BE PRESCRIBED**

Your diagnosis is achieved through a consultation process which uses techniques of interrogation, observation and palpation (examination through the sense of touch). These are the three means of access to knowledge – that is, *pratyaksha* (cognitive sensory knowledge, inference or judgement), and *aptopadesh* (use of past experience, research or textual evidence).

Before technology made its inroads into the field of medicine, it was only through the doctor–patient relationship and the information provided by the patient that proper diagnosis and decisions regarding treatment could be made. This does not mean that the ayurvedic consultation is an anachronism in today's hi-tech world. Properly utilized, the practitioner's five senses, combined with sound reflective and inferential skills, will enable them to elicit all the information needed to make a correct diagnosis and to make decisions about treatment and management of the patient's condition. Above all, the objective will be to re-balance your doshas, not merely to relieve the symptoms.

Ayurvedic examination

Diagnosis in ayurveda depends mainly on your prakruti (physical constitution) and any imbalances in your body. These imbalances primarily relate to the three doshas of vata, pitta and kapha; however, in the case of a fully established disease, imbalances relating to agni (digestive fire), body tissues and waste materials are also significant. Diagnosis is facilitated through the process of examination, which has three clear goals:

- Assessing the quality of your life and the quantity of your life span
- Assessing the aggravation or decrease related to doshas in terms of quality and quantity
- Assessing your strength, resistance and immunity

These threefold goals need to be achieved through a twofold approach:

- Examination of the patient – this is known as the tenfold examination
- Examination of the physical manifestations of the disease – known as the eightfold examination

The tenfold examination

A physical examination in an ayurvedic consultation consists of questioning, observation and touching the patient. The ten factors associated with your normal physical and mental state are assessed first. This is known as the tenfold examination, and includes:

- Prakruti (physical constitution)
- Psychological constitution (mental traits and personality traits)
- Condition of tissues and nutritional status
- Physical build
- Height, weight, biometry or the size and proportions of your body
- Adaptability (for example, food intolerances and allergies)
- Digestive capacity
- Capacity for exercise
- Age/stage of life
- Place of birth and place of residence

This type of questioning helps the practitioner to build a picture of the history of your illness, including past, current and chronic illnesses or symptoms, as well as your personal history, your family history and, in the case of women, your menstrual and obstetric history.

The eightfold examination

When you see an ayurvedic practitioner, the eightfold examination is to assess the degree of disorder of your doshas, the seven body tissues, and waste products. This is collectively known as *vikriti*, and it helps to give the practitioner an overview of your general condition and the nature and extent of your illness. During the examination, the following eight things are considered:

- Pulse
- Urine
- Faecal matter
- Tongue
- Voice and speech
- Touch, skin and tactile sense
- Eyes and vision
- General appearance

Where necessary, the following will also be included on the list of things to be examined:

- Semen
- Breast milk
- Sputum
- Hair
- Blood
- Menstrual blood
- Perspiration
- Fingernails
- Saliva

Our body and its waste products reflect the state of balance of our body. Looking at these things can help to identify any imbalances in the doshas.

COLOUR

In ayurveda, each of the three doshas is associated with particular colours:

- Vata – brown or black
- Pitta – yellow, green or red
- Kapha – pale colours or white

These colours are extremely helpful in establishing which of the three doshas in your body is in excess. Colour changes can be seen on your tongue and in your stools, urine, skin and phlegm.

PULSE EXAMINATION

The initial pulse examination should always be done early in the morning, after you have woken up and tended to your morning ablutions, but before you eat anything. This gives the base or indicating pulse for your prakruti (see pages 28–34). Your pulse can then be checked at different times of the day to see whether there are any doshic features or imbalances.

When your pulse is being taken, the radial pulse below the thumb (on the right hand for males, and the left hand for females) should be examined using three fingers (second, middle and ring finger). Both you and the practitioner examining your pulse should be seated comfortably, and you need to be monitored for at least a minute.

- Vata pulse is felt as very rapid, shallow and irregular in any of the three finger positions
- Pitta pulse is felt as a strong, regular beat in any of the three finger positions
- Kapha pulse is felt as slow, deep and weak in any of the three finger positions
- If a vata pulse (fast and irregular) is felt in any other place than the first finger position (vata position), vata is unbalanced
- If a pitta pulse (strong and regular) is felt in any other place than the middle finger position (pitta position), pitta is unbalanced

- If a kapha pulse (slow and deep) is felt in any other place than the last finger position (kapha position), kapha is unbalanced
- An increase in vata makes the pulse even faster at the vata position, while decreased vata slows it
- An increase in pitta makes the pulse stronger than normal at the pitta position, while decreased pitta makes it weaker at this position
- An increase in kapha makes the pulse stronger than usual at the kapha position, whereas it is very slow and deep if kapha is decreased

URINE EXAMINATION

You will be asked to provide a urine sample, as well as answer questions from the practitioner. For the purposes of midstream examination, urine must be collected in the morning, in a clean container.

Your urine should be clear without much foam, but you should also bear in mind that eating certain foods can affect your urine with no ill effects. Asparagus, cabbage, cauliflower and garlic can all give your urine a distinctive smell. Abnormal observations are:

- Muddy, thick urine
- Scanty urine
- Dark yellow urine
- Whitish, foamy urine
- Dull-coloured urine
- Reddish urine
- Strong odorous urine

STOOL EXAMINATION

Your stools should be neither too hard nor too soft (about the consistency of a ripe banana). They should float rather than sink in water and should not have a foul odour. You should be able to pass faeces once or twice a day without straining. The practitioner will be looking for any of the following abnormalities:

- Hard, dry stool
- Greenish liquid stool
- Mucus in stool
- Grey or blackish stool
- Whitish sticky stool

TONGUE EXAMINATION

The tongue mirrors what is happening inside your stomach and body. Tongue diagnosis can be very subtle, and ayurvedic practitioners develop this skill over many years.

In ayurveda, cleaning your tongue every morning is an important part of daily routine (see pages 69–70). Normally, you should use a metal tongue scraper to clean off any accumulation on the tongue – this stimulates your taste buds.

The actual shape and colour of the tongue are indicators of your basic constitution (prakruti). A thin, trembling, pale tongue shows a vata constitution, while a medium, reddish tongue is due to a pitta constitution. A thick, rounded, pale and white tongue is indicative of kapha.

For practical purposes, the whole tongue is divided into three portions: the rear relates to vata; the middle to pitta; and the front to kapha. Any abnormality evident on the various parts of the tongue such as lumps, depressions, growths or a build-up of waste directly indicates an imbalance in the respective dosha it represents.

A healthy tongue should be pink, clear and have lustre. Examine the actual colour and texture of your tongue to see if you have any of these signs:

- Dry, rough tongue
- Cracks in the tongue
- Brownish tongue
- Reddish tongue
- Burning tongue
- Furrowed tongue
- Bluish tongue
- Blackish tongue
- Yellow-green tongue
- Mucus on the tongue
- White coating on the tongue
- Painful bristles on the tongue

VOICE AND SPEECH EXAMINATION

Your tone of voice and speech patterns are also indications of your prakruti. For example, a low, monotonous voice tends to represent vata, while speaking in a precise, clear manner indicates pitta. A deep, measured voice is usually indicative of people with a kapha prakruti.

SKIN EXAMINATION

If your skin is healthy, it will be smooth with uniform temperature all over the body. Abnormal changes are:

- Low skin temperature
- Rough, dry skin
- Hot skin
- Cold hands and feet
- Hot hands and feet
- Cold, oily skin

EYE EXAMINATION

Any imbalance in the doshas can also be seen in your eyes. The practitioner will look for the following:

- Rust-coloured eyes
- Smoky eyes
- Dull eye movements
- Drooping upper eyelid
- Pink or red eyes
- Yellowish eyes
- Burning

FINGERNAIL EXAMINATION

Healthy fingernails are smooth and well shaped. Longitudinal striations in nails, bitten nails, a bump at the end of a nail, or a parrot beak at end of a nail, all indicate an imbalance in the doshas.

PERSPIRATION EXAMINATION

Your perspiration should be colour and odour free, although there may be temporary smells due to foods you have recently eaten. Observations might include:

• Excessive perspiration
• Malodorous perspiration
• Perspiration in cool weather

LIPS EXAMINATION

Evaluation of doshas can also be made through the appearance of your lips, for example:

• Dry, rough lips indicate vata
• Inflamed patches are a sign of pitta
• Moderately dry lips mean kapha

All these observations will need to be done by the practitioner in a particular way and at a particular time.

Examination of the disease

After the tenfold and eightfold examinations have been carried out, the next step will be examination of the state of the disease. There are five things that your ayurvedic physician will look at here:

• Aetiology, or the causes of the disease
• Early symptoms
• Signs and symptoms
• Alleviating factors
• Pathogenesis, or the development of the disease

Ayurvedic texts such as *Madhav Nidan* and the *Charaka Samhita* describe these factors for each disease in great detail.

The principles of treatment

In ayurveda, disease is seen as the result of the three doshas being out of equilibrium, while health is the result of their being in equilibrium. Diseases, in turn, are of two kinds: organic (arising from the body itself) and traumatic (arising from external causes). The seats for these two types of diseases are the physical body and the mind.

The doshas (vata, kapha and pitta), the body's tissues (*dhatus*) and its wastes (*malas*) are the fundamental roots of our bodies throughout our life span. Our digestive fire (*agni*) has its own influences (see pages 74 and 78–9). It is present in our body tissues, and any increase or decrease in its quantity, quality or functions gives rise to a corresponding increase or decrease in the body tissues. Our body tissues are interlinked, so that any increase or decrease in one of our tissues will cause the same condition in successive ones.

If any one of the doshas becomes unbalanced, this will have an unbalancing effect on our blood and other tissues. Both the doshas and the body tissues affect the balance of our bodies' waste products, which in turn affect their channels of elimination. It is from these unbalanced or degraded channels of elimination that disease develops.

Diseases arising from specific causative factors, such as food, particular activities or thoughts and emotions, and that bring about an increase of in any of the doshas, are said to be doshic diseases. Those arising without any apparent or idiopathic cause are known as karmaja diseases (that is, they are born out of the effects of any bad actions committed in previous lives). Those diseases that are severe in both onset and manifestation are said to be a combination of both. Doshic diseases are generally cured if they are treated with foods, drugs and activities that possess the opposite qualities to the unbalanced dosha. The second group of diseases, those related to karma, are cured by modifying your actions so that you lead a more spiritually healthy life. The final group, where diseases are the result of both doshic imbalances and karmic actions, require the combination of both approaches.

The treatment of a disease or imbalance requires a proper assessment of both the patient and the disease. The ayurvedic physician always has the final decision.

As a rule, before any treatment is undertaken, your ayurvedic physician should have acquired information about the following:

• The condition of the three doshas
• Any imbalances in, or problems with, associated tissues, waste products or metabolites
• Your lifestyle and living conditions
• Your physical and immunological strength
• The state of your digestion and metabolism
• Your individual constitution
• Your age
• Your mind/psyche and psychological strength
• Any allergies that you suffer from

- Your dietary and food habits
- The stage of your disease

The definition of treatment

Any approach toward the attempted cure of a disease is considered treatment (*chikitsa*). In ayurveda, treatment is regarded as a complex operation involving the best of the four arms of therapeutic practice – the physician, herbal medicines and diet, the attendant or nurse and the individual patient. It is also important to note that successful relief of symptoms alone is not considered as treatment in ayurveda.

Treatment of the doshas

According to ayurveda, the doshas are the chief cause of all diseases. Even the disturbances found in body tissues and waste products result from imbalances of the doshas. Understanding the principles of balancing the doshas is therefore of prime importance to an ayurvedic physician. This is mainly achieved by changes to your diet, activities, thoughts and perceptions, and through drugs and/or therapies.

Doshas cause imbalance by either increasing (*vridhi*) or decreasing (*kshaya*) in terms of quantity, quality or both, as well as in terms of how they function. The increase of a dosha can be defined by the decrease of its opposite qualities, and the increase of similar qualities. The opposite is true when a dosha decreases. Therefore, when increased, the doshas produce their respective features (signs and symptoms) depending upon the strength of the increase, and when decreased, they cast off their normal features.

The increase and decrease of the doshas are influenced by the avoidance of foods that are disliked and the indulgence of foods that are desired, provided that such foods are not unsuitable. Doshas that are increased or decreased generally produce a desire for foods that are dissimilar and similar, respectively. For example, if you are suffering from aggravated vata, you will crave foods that do not produce this dosha, such as sweet things. If vata is diminished, you will crave vata-producing foods, such as chickpeas.

A more detailed explanation of various approaches and treatments to be undertaken in the case of vata increase, pitta increase and kapha increase is listed in the box, right, and on the following pages.

The different treatments prescribed for each individual dosha may be combined appropriately in conditions involving the combination of two or three doshas.

Dosha treatment guidelines

TREATMENT OF INCREASED VATA DOSHA
- Oil and fats (*snehana*)
- Perspiration (*swedana*)
- Diet consisting of oily, hot, sweet, sour and salty foods (for example, spicy foods, citrus fruits, dates)
- Oil massage (*abyanga*)
- Kneading the body (*mardana*)
- Wrapping the body with cloth (*vestanam*)
- Taking a stern or firm approach
- Bathing/pouring of medicated water
- Alcohol/wine
- Medicated enemas (*basti*)/oil enemas (*tailanuvaasana*)

TREATMENT OF INCREASED PITTA DOSHA
- Drinking ghee (*snehana*)
- Purgation – sweet and cold herbs (*virechana*)
- Diet and drugs – sweet, bitter and astringent (for example, rice, coconut, Brussels sprouts, asparagus)
- Use of perfumes that are pleasing and cooling
- Garlands around the neck and chest
- Wearing gems
- Applying the paste of herbs such as camphor, sandalwood and vetiver
- Listening to pleasant music
- Enjoying a cool breeze
- Enjoying the company of friends and family
- Ideally, living in a house with fountains, parks, ponds and gardens
- Drinking milk

TREATMENT OF INCREASED KAPHA DOSHA
- Emesis – strong (*vamana*)
- Purgation – strong (*virechana*)
- Diet consisting of dry, non-fatty, slightly penetrating, hot, pungent, bitter and astringent foods in small quantities (for example, spices such as black pepper and cumin, garlic, apples)
- Aged wines/alcohol
- Indulging in sex
- Not oversleeping and not sleeping during the day
- Varied exercise
- Mindfulness or examining your actions
- Dry massage
- Drinking soups
- Honey
- Drugs that reduce fat
- Medicated smoking (herbal cigarettes)
- Fasting
- Medicated gargling
- Avoiding a sedentary lifestyle

Generally, the treatment for a vata-pitta combination will be similar to the seasonal regimen for summer; for that of kapha-vata, it will be similar to the seasonal regimen for spring; and, for the kapha-pitta combination, the treatment will be similar to the seasonal regimen for autumn (see pages 70–1).

Where each of the three doshas are unbalanced simultaneously, the most powerful should be controlled without opposing the remaining doshas.

TREATMENT OF THE DOSHAS ACCORDING TO DIFFERENT STAGES

It is always preferable to treat the doshas in their accumulation stage, when they show an increase at their own sites (see the pathways of disease on page 42). Treatment at this stage is easy and effective, and can restore balance perfectly. During the aggravation stage, when increased doshas spread from their own sites to other sites in your body and affect the functioning of the other doshas, they should be handled carefully, with a judicious assessment of the strength of each dosha. The dominant dosha should be pacified first, without opposing the other less powerful doshas. This is just one of the reasons why it is important that you consult a qualified ayurvedic doctor.

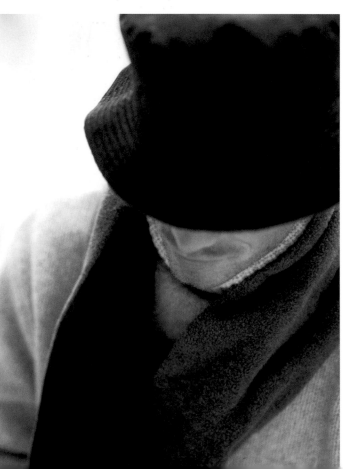

How to balance the doshas

VATA
- Go to bed early
- Eat meals at the same time every day
- Ensure regular elimination
- Keep warm in cold weather
- Drink plenty of warm liquids
- Favour sweet, sour and salty foods

Vata needs calming and a regular routine

PITTA
- Avoid extreme heat or exposure to the sun
- Abstain from alcohol and smoking
- Avoid overactivity
- Finish work on time and avoid stressful deadlines
- Avoid skipping meals, especially lunch
- Favour sweet, astringent and bitter foods
- Avoid spicy, sour and salty foods

Pitta needs cooling and moderation

KAPHA
- Avoid excessive rest and oversleeping
- Get plenty of exercise
- Seek out variety in life
- Keep warm in cold, wet weather
- Favour spicy, bitter and astringent foods
- Avoid eating heavy, oily foods

Kapha needs warming and stimulation

Treatment of imbalance in tissues and waste products

The tissues and waste products or metabolites also undergo imbalance, which is, of course, the after effect of dosha imbalance. When tissues, waste products or metabolites increase or decrease from their normal state, they give rise to various symptoms of disease. An increase of body fluids, lymph and blood, may require purgation, known as *virechana*; in the case of muscle tissue, it may be necessary to undergo surgery, cauterization and thermal cautery. For diseases arising due to fatty tissue or lipids, an approach similar to the management of obesity is necessary. Bone diseases subside through the administration of herbal enemas (*basti*) consisting of milk and ghee processed with bitter herbs, such as golden seal.

left **DRESSING WARMLY IN COLD, WET WEATHER IS IMPORTANT IN KEEPING BOTH VATA DOSHA AND KAPHA DOSHA IN BALANCE**

The natural art of balancing doshas

Health and disease are two inevitable states of being. Ayurveda relates both health and disease to the balance or imbalance of doshas. Balance leads to health, imbalance to disease. Every human activity, experience and thought influences your doshas, as do food, the seasons, your age and your genetic imprint. The ayurvedic way of positive lifestyle, diet, sex and relationships, is designed to keep your doshas balanced and healthy, so that you can maintain and preserve your health, night and day, every day, throughout your life.

When it comes to illness and disease, the undeniable link between mind and body cannot be overlooked, and no healing process is complete without addressing the imbalances on this most fundamental level. Unfortunately, the single-shot approach of allopathic medicine (the method of treating disease by the use of agents that produce effects opposite to those of the disease) occasionally carries over into the practice of ayurvedic medicine. Herbs, nutritional supplements and single-chemical herbal drugs are often used to alleviate symptoms or treat diseases without any attempt to locate and address the deeper levels of the problem. This ignores one of the fundamental tenets of ayurveda – that mind, body and spirit must be treated holistically. For the process of healing to be complete, an ayurvedic physician must be able to activate and harness all aspects of his or her intelligence involved in the transformation of consciousness into matter. Indeed, ayurveda provides a different channel for maintaining physiological balance, and emotional and mental wellbeing. Each of the ayurvedic therapeutic interventions and approaches should be individually tailored to address your unique psycho-physiological make-up. The authentic ayurvedic approach usually encompasses the following:

- Treat the person as a whole. Body and mind are inseparable in a living person and the cure should always address the psychosomatic factors. Body structures and functions cannot be studied or treated in isolation.
- Give the drug as a whole. In its naturally occurring form, each substance (dietary or drug) is like a little packet of nature's intelligence which our bodies can use to counterbalance disruptive influences from the environment. Isolation and administration of active principles from plants effect the cure quickly, but can cause side effects or lead to complications. According to Charaka, 'Ideal treatment is that which cures the disease and does not cause any other (iatrogenic) disease.'
- It is also important that have a strong physique and mind, and kind heart, so that your immune system is strengthened. In fact, it is the body's immune system which is responsible for most cures. The strength achieved through a robust immune system also makes the individual healthy and happy, and useful to society, the nation and the world. This gives meaning to life and lends decency to living – important facets of the purity of mind, body and spirit which ayurvedic living seeks to achieve.
- The body is more important than the microbe. Stress is placed on increasing the resistance of the body, rather than killing the microbes. Humans are miniatures of the cosmos. Humankind has been studied in relation to its surroundings and environment, and there is reciprocity between them, so both should be treated simultaneously.

Doshas – the root causes

The common aim of treatment that works on the level of the body is to purify the body and restore balance to each of the three doshas. The doshas are the root cause of all illness, physical or mental, in ayurveda.

A knowledge of the doshas and their relative state of balance or imbalance presents a unique means of monitoring the state of the body and detecting imbalances long before they show up as symptoms of disease. Additionally, if symptoms are already present, assessing the dosha imbalances in your body enables the physician to pinpoint the underlying cause of the symptoms or disease. Therapies can then be applied that address the physiological imbalance created by the imbalance of the doshas, rather than merely the symptoms themselves. This links to the ayurvedic principles of prevention rather than cure, and treating the body as a whole instead of disease in isolation. The primary focus for ayurvedic healing is balancing the unbalanced doshas through a combination of food, lifestyle, mental exercises, herbal drugs and medicines, and detoxification and rejuvenation therapies.

Purification techniques and ayurvedic remedies

Therapeutic treatments have an important role to play in ayurveda. Carefully targeted interventions are crucial in eliminating dosha and sub-dosha imbalances, especially when symptoms of disease are present. Even for a person of basic good health, therapeutic treatments provide a vehicle for moving further towards the health end of the health–disease spectrum.

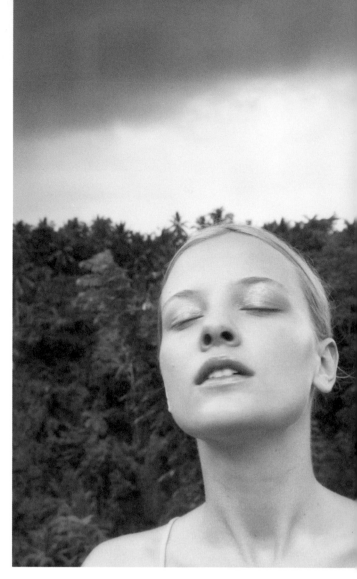

PANCHAKARMA

The ayurvedic techniques for purifying, eliminating and balancing the physiology of the doshas are known as *panchakarma*. Translated as 'the five actions', panchakarma is a medley of treatments that aim to clear impurities from the body and balance the doshas. The methodical approach followed in panchakarma first dislodges the toxins (*ama*) from the body's cells, then removes the increased dosha from the diseased site, before flushing it out through the organs of elimination – the sweat glands, the intestines and the urinary tract. The main focus of panchakarma is to clear the bodily channels, or *srotas*. There are innumerable such channels in our bodies, and clearing the ama and unbalanced doshas helps to maintain a proper metabolic equilibrium in the body and also facilitates a quicker, more complete healing process.

The nature of the panchakarma treatment varies from one individual to another, but in general there are three main steps involved:

• Preparatory purification processes
• The main treatment
• Aftercare

The preparatory purification processes include the administration of oil, ghee and fats for a period of three, five or seven days, followed by oil massage and sweating therapies, collectively known as *snehana* and *swedana*. You should initially undergo a process of taking digestive and carminative herbs to help to detoxify your system. Panchakarma is only carried out once your body is free from ama.

After the initial purification steps, you will undergo the main purification therapies (see pages 57–62).

Note of caution

Bloodletting, used to purify the blood, is traditionally part of panchakarma. It is commonly adopted in surgical practice only. Bloodletting is even coming back into favour in some areas of Western medicine through the use of leeches. It should be noted, however, that bloodletting is illegal in the USA. Also, as with all elements of panchakarma, it should only be carried out by a fully qualified ayurvedic physician with the minimum of a university degree and five years' experience.

When your main panchakarma treatment is complete, you will be required to rest and to adhere to a strict dietary regime to bring you back to your original diet and activity level. This process, known as *samsarjana karma*, takes between three to seven days.

A typical panchakarma treatment takes about two hours per day. The length of the course of treatment can vary from three days to two weeks, depending on the condition of your individual constitution. For maximum effect, you should receive panchakarma several times a year, preferably at the change of the seasons. Pilot studies have shown that panchakarma retards the ageing process and improves both mental and physical health by reducing the risk of neurovascular, neuromuscular and cardiovascular complications. People who have undergone these treatments report greater wellbeing and emotional stability; increased energy, vitality and youthfulness; better digestion; an improvement in physical symptoms of disease; and a general feeling of relaxation and serenity.

Ayurvedic pharmacology

The ayurvedic materia medica contains knowledge of thousands of medicinal plants and herbal and mineral mixtures. Some of these are mild in their action, while others have more potent and specific effects. Among the mild medicinal substance are several well-known spices and herbs, which can easily be adopted as part of the home pharmacy. Turmeric, for example, is an excellent blood purifier and also useful for eliminating excess mucus from a sore throat. Ginger is an excellent digestive – nothing fans the digestive fire as much as a piece of fresh ginger, with a pinch of rock salt, before a meal. The cooling effect of aloe vera juice is helpful for pitta disorders, while liquorice tea is good for balancing vata. The curative powers of these standard kitchen ingredients are part of traditional folklore. However, the dosage and administration of the complex compound formulations of ayurveda require a better knowledge of the pharmacological basis of ayurvedic medicine and should be left to a qualified doctor. The basis of ayurvedic therapeutics rests on five well-defined pharmacological principles:

Taste (rasa) – This has already been discussed in detail (see pages 36–9). If you taste the drug with your tongue, its action readily follows. This does not mean that the drug acts through taste alone.

Physical or biological property – There are 20 in total, or ten pairs of opposites (see page 36). Of these, six are therapeutically important: oiliness, coldness, heaviness, dryness, heat and lightness. The first three are anabolic; the others are catabolic. Anabolic and catabolic approaches lie at the root of ayurvedic therapy (see page 78).

Post-digestive effect of the drug (vipaka) – The six tastes of drugs or food are broken down into three effects after digestion. Sweet and salty tastes are converted into sweet vipaka. Sour remains sour after digestion, and bitter, pungent and astringent tastes change to pungent vipaka. A sweet post-digestive taste influences kapha dosha, a sour post-digestive taste influences pitta dosha and a pungent post-digestive taste influences vata.

Potency of a drug (veerya) – This is generally that quality of a drug (out of the 10 pairs described above) with a specific action. The active principle of a drug is known as veerya and there are considered to be two types: cold (sita) potency and hot (ushna) potency. Sita potency retards, stops, slows or blocks, while ushna accelerates, moves or speeds action in the body.

Isomerism (prabhava) – Drugs that are apparently similar may have entirely different actions. While their atomic number may be the same, their configuration differs and hence also their actions.

Ayurvedic physicians well versed in these five pillars of pharmacology (if they have acquired proper clinical skill and judgement) can use anything available to them, as a food or drug, to heal. The simplicity of ayurveda is that it uses the same yardsticks to evaluate both food and drugs.

The classical ayurvedic texts list the following benefits for panchakarma:

- Improvement in agni (digestive fire, or metabolism)
- Relief from disease
- The restoration of normal health
- Clearer senses, mind and intellect
- Improved complexion
- Increased strength
- Improved nourishment of the body
- Increased fertility
- Reduction in the effects of ageing
- Increased longevity and happiness

Panchakarma is a double-edged sword. Its value as a therapeutic intervention can only be achieved if it is administered under the guidance of an appropriately qualified ayurvedic specialist. If it is mismanaged, it could greatly endanger your health. In fact, one of the causes listed for many diseases in ayurveda is the abuse of panchakarma.

DRUG THERAPY

Drug therapy is the basis of ayurvedic management of many diseases acute or chronic. Ayurvedic medicines are derived from plants, herbs or minerals. They can be administered as single ingredients or combined in ways that enhance their therapeutic value. More than 15,000 formulations are described in the ayurvedic pharmacopoeia. Many of these are still prescribed today and are successful in treating various illnesses.

OTHER HEALING THERAPIES OF AYURVEDA

In the West, other ayurvedic healing treatments such as massage, shirodhara and oil baths are becoming popular. People often misunderstand these to be part of panchakarma. Although they are all ayurvedic healing therapies, they are not purification processes in themselves. They are often involved in the preparation process for panchakarma or, in certain situations, are done independently to prevent illness. These therapies come under either snehana or swedana in ayurvedic healing. Sometimes they do both together, as in the case of oil baths, *pizzhichil* or *sonvangadhara*.

An introduction to panchakarma

Health is the condition when the doshas are in their 'natural rhythm'; this is a state of order. When this rhythm is lost, it is known as disease and this is a state of disorder. Living in a state of order is at the heart of ayurveda, and setting any disorder back into order is called healing (*chikitsa* or *upakrama*).

Doshas cannot be identified separately when they are each in balance. However, in a diseased condition particular symptoms and signs are manifested which are specific to a particular dosha. These symptoms and signs denote malfunctioning of the body, its organs, tissues or a cell. The purpose of any treatment in ayurveda is to keep the doshas in their natural equilibrium or rhythm. Generally, this is achieved through a cleansing process (*samshodana*), restoration achieved by palliative care (*samshamana*) and treating or eliminating the causative factors (*nidana parivartana*). Of the three, the cleansing process is considered to be the most important, as it eliminates aggravated or unbalanced doshas from the body and also eradicates the disease permanently, without leaving any chance for relapse. This is where the concept of panchakarma comes into its own.

What is panchakarma?

In Sanskrit, *pancha* means 'five' and *karma* means 'actions'. Thus, panchakarma is a group of five actions, or therapies. Panchakarma is also a synonym for samshodana, or cleansing. All the ancient ayurvedic texts describe these five different types of therapy in detail, but the term panchakarma is only used frequently by Charaka. There is also some debate regarding exactly which five therapies should be included under this heading.

According to Charaka, the five therapies are:

- Induced herbal emesis (*vamana*)
- Induced herbal purgation (*virechana*)
- Rectal administration of decoction enemas (*niruha*, or *asthapana*)
- Rectal administration of oil enemas (*anuvasana*)
- Nasal administration of herbal oils, powders or juices (*sirovirechana*, or *nasya*)

According to Sushruta, the five elemental therapies of panchakarma are:

- Emesis therapy (*vamana*) for kapha elimination
- Herbal purgation (*virechana*) for pitta elimination
- Herbal enemas (*basti*) for balancing vata
- Nasal herbal drops (*nasya*) for doshas above the head and neck region (irrespective of the type of dosha)
- Bloodletting (*raktamokshana*)

What is its basic concept?

As already discussed, the primary control of all biological activities lies in the three doshas. These doshas are, in turn, under the influence of day and night, the seasons, climate, food and a person's physical and mental activities. This is why the doshas exhibit changes such as accumulation, aggravation (increase) and spread. These changes take place inside your body unnoticed. However, if this physiological process is disturbed due to various causes, the doshas reach a noticeable state of aggravation. As a result of this, they start to move out of their normal sites, circulating throughout your body. Here they join with weaker tissues or metabolic wastes. This causes disturbances in the various channels of the body, resulting in various diseases.

These unbalanced doshas move from primary or internal disease channels to secondary, outer or deeper disease channels, making it still more complicated and difficult to eliminate them from your body. When an unbalanced dosha has moved to a deeper level, simple pacification will provide only temporary relief, masking the symptoms. The unbalanced dosha awaits a suitable time and weaker site to manifest once again as a relapse, or as an entirely different disease. Ayurveda therefore advocates that those excessively aggravated doshas, those which have moved from the primary to the secondary channels of the body, should be eliminated quickly, before they cause further damage. To achieve this elimination, it is necessary that the doshas be brought back to the gut, from where they can be eliminated easily and effectively by panchakarma.

Poorva karma

Poorva karma, the preparatory purification stage of panchakarma, is a prerequisite for panchakarma. It not only prepares you for elimination therapy, but is also necessary to achieve the best results.

According to ayurveda, if any dosha is associated with ama (toxins), elimination should never be attempted. Therefore, before you proceed to panchakarma therapy, an ayurvedic physician *must* assess you to see

right **MASSAGE WITH OILS IS USED TO CLEANSE YOUR BODY OF IMPURITIES THROUGH YOUR SKIN IN PREPARATION FOR THE DEEPER DETOXIFICATION OF PANCHAKARMA ITSELF**

whether there is any ama present in your body. If this is the case, you should be treated for this first. Therefore, as a first step, you will be prescribed deepan (digestive) and pachan (carminative) herbs for about a week, to digest ama and make your agni (digestive fire) function normally. Your stools should be checked for abnormalities during this stage. If they float normally and your tongue is clear, it is an indication that there is no ama and your agni is functioning well. Only then should further treatments be undertaken. There should be no rush to start elimination therapies immediately.

The first step is snehana. It is essential that you have oil therapy before each panchakarma session until the physician believes you are exhibiting symptoms of what is known as being properly oleated.

Oil therapy is given both internally and externally, and can be administered through different kinds of foods, or through enemas and massage. It is further classified into various types. In poorva karma, internal oil therapy is used initially and then followed by external oil therapy. The internal therapy is continued until you show signs of proper saturation of oils in the body. There are two methods used here:

• Pure oil or ghee
• Processed herbal oil or ghee, sometimes along with food

It is for the physician to judge the method of administration on the basis of your constitution and condition. There are about 24 different varieties of internal oil therapy. It is therefore essential that the ayurvedic practitioner knows when oil therapy should and should not be used. They should also clearly advise you on the type of food, activities, thoughts and behaviour necessary during this period. Commonly, internal oil therapy takes three, five or seven days, depending on your prakruti and dosha. External oil therapy takes the form of massage. You will undertake massage using herbal oils designed to cleanse your body of impurities through your skin. This can be either a full body massage or a head massage.

Poorva karma also involves swedana (sweating therapy). It always follows oil therapy and, depending on the form of the main panchakarma therapy, is done over one, two, three or more days. Swedana is always administered alongside external oil therapy, or massage, and also involves the use of medicinal herbs.

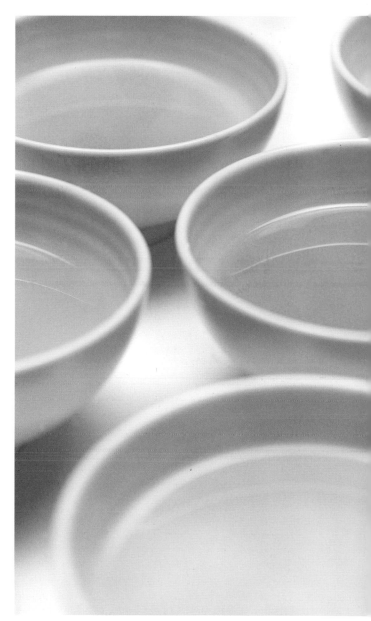

Pradhana karma

The five main purification methods used in the main treatment of panchakarma are known as *pradhana karma*. One, or a combination of the following, may be used to treat you after your ayurvedic physician has made a complete diagnosis and your body has been cleared of ama through poorva karma:

• Therapeutic vomiting or emesis therapy – vamana
• Purgation therapy – virechana
• Enema therapy – basti
• Nasal therapy (elimination of toxins through the nose) – nasya
• Detoxification of the blood – raktamoksha

EMESIS THERAPY

When there is congestion in the lungs causing repeated attacks of bronchitis, colds, coughs or asthma, the ayurvedic treatment is vamana, to eliminate the kapha causing the excess mucus. After the oil and sweating therapies, you will be given three or four glasses of liquorice or salt water to drink, then vomiting is stimulated by rubbing your tongue. Often, this also releases repressed emotions which have been held in the kapha areas of the lungs and stomach, along with the accumulated dosha.

It is likely that congestion, breathlessness and wheezing will disappear and your sinuses will become clear. Therapeutic vomiting is also indicated in chronic asthma, diabetes, chronic cold, lymphatic congestion, chronic indigestion and oedema (swelling).

Before emesis therapy is administered, oil massage and sweating therapy must be carried out. One to three days prior to emesis therapy, you will be asked to drink a cup of recommended oil two or three times a day until your stools become oily, or until you feel nauseated. You should also eat a kaphagenic diet (see page 77) to aggravate kapha in your system.

Emesis therapy should be given early in the morning (when kapha is dominant). Eating basmati rice and yogurt with plenty of salt early in the morning will further aggravate kapha in your stomach. Applying heat to your chest and back will liquefy the kapha.

You will be asked to sit on a straight-backed chair and drink the concoction of liquorice and honey, or salt water in a calm manner. This preparation is measured and recorded, so that after the procedure the amount of vomit resulting from the decoction can be determined. The degree of success in this treatment is determined by:

- The number of times you vomit (eight is maximum, six medium, four minimum)
- The amount you vomit

After emesis therapy, resting, fasting and smoking certain herbal cigarettes are recommended. If emesis therapy is administered properly, you will be able to breathe freely and feel a lightness in your chest. Your thinking will be clear, as will your voice, and you will have developed a healthy appetite. All symptoms of congestion should disappear.

After undergoing emesis therapy in the morning, you should fast until 5 pm, then eat kitchari (see page 122) with ghee. You should also drink cumin, coriander,

Indications for emesis therapy

- All kapha-type disorders
- Pitta headache, dizziness and nausea
- Need to release blocked emotions
- Respiratory congestion
- Bronchitis
- Chronic cold
- Sinus congestion
- Kapha-type asthma

Contraindications

- People below the age of 12 or over 65
- Menstruation
- Premenstrual period (one week prior)
- Pregnancy
- Emaciation
- Delicate or sensitive person with too much fear, grief or anxiety
- Hypoglycaemia
- Vata prakruti
- Vata diseases
- Heart diseases
- During vata season
- Acute fever
- Diarrhoea
- Obesity

ginger and fennel tea (in equal proportions). Steep in hot water and drink with one teaspoon of honey. Alternatively, honey and lime tea is also recommended. It should be made using one teaspoon of honey and one teaspoon of lime juice to a cup hot of water.

PURGATION THERAPY

When excess bile or pitta is secreted and accumulates in the gall bladder, liver and small intestine, it tends to result in rashes, skin inflammation, acne, chronic attacks of fever, biliary vomiting, nausea and jaundice. Ayurvedic literature recommends the administration of virechana (therapeutic purgation or a therapeutic laxative) for these conditions. Purging is facilitated with senna leaves, flax seed, psyllium husks or triphala in a combination that is appropriate for the individual person.

Senna-leaf tea is a mild laxative, but is not used if you have a vata constitution, as it can create griping pain. This is because its action aggravates peristaltic movement in the large intestine.

An effective laxative for vata or pitta constitutions is a glass of hot milk to which two teaspoons ghee (clarified butter) have been added. This laxative, taken at bedtime, will help to relieve excess pitta, which causes bile disturbance in the body. In fact, purgatives can completely cure the problem of excess pitta.

Daily restrictions must be carefully observed when purgatives are used and, as with all elements of panchakarma, they should be taken only under the care of a qualified ayurvedic physician. You should not eat foods that will aggravate the predominant dosha or cause any of the three doshas to become unbalanced.

Substances used: Senna, prunes, bran, flaxseed husk, dandelion root, psyllium seed, cow's milk, salt, castor oil, raisins, mango juice, triphala.

Indications for purgation therapy

- Allergic rashes
- Skin inflammation
- Acne, dermatitis, eczema
- Chronic fever
- Ascites
- Biliary vomiting
- Jaundice
- Urinary disorder
- Enlargement of the spleen
- Internal worms
- Burning sensation in the eyes
- Inflammation of the eyes
- Conjunctivitis
- Gout

Contraindications

- Low digestive fire (agni)
- Acute fever
- Diarrhoea
- Severe constipation
- Bleeding from the rectum or lung cavities
- Foreign body in the stomach
- Following enema
- Emaciation or weakness
- Prolapsed rectum
- Alcoholism
- Dehydration
- Childhood
- Old age
- Ulcerative colitis

ENEMA THERAPY

Vata's predominant site is the colon or large intestine. Basti enema therapy involves introducing concoctions of sesame oil together with herbal preparations in a liquid medium into the rectum. Enema therapy is the most effective treatment for vata disorders, although many enemas over a prescribed period of time are usually required. It relieves constipation, distention, chronic fever, colds, sexual disorders, kidney stones, heart pain, backache, sciatica and other pains in the joints. Many other vata disorders such as gout, arthritis, rheumatism, muscle spasms and headaches may also be treated with enema therapy.

Vata is the primary aetiological factor in the manifestation of diseases. It is the motivating force behind the elimination and retention of faeces, urine, bile and other excreta. Vata is mainly located in the large intestine, but bone tissue is also a site for vata. The mucus membrane of the colon is related to the outer covering of the bones (periosteum), which nourishes the bones. Therefore, any medication given rectally goes into the deeper tissues, such as bones, and corrects vata disorders.

There are eight main types of enema therapy, each with its own indications and contra-indications.

- Oil enema (*Anuvasana*) – used in pure vata disorders and when you are experiencing excess hunger or dryness related to vata imbalances.
- Decoction enema (*Niruha-asthapana*) – used for evacuation of vata, nervous diseases, gastro-intestinal vata conditions, gout, certain fevers, unconsciousness, certain urinary conditions, appetite stimulation, pain, hyperacidity and heart diseases, among other conditions.
- Urethral in males or vaginal in females (*Uttara basti*) – used for selected semen and ovulation disorders and for some problems involving painful urination or bladder infections. This treatment should not be used if you have diabetes.
- Daily oil enema (*Matra basti*) – used if you are run down or emaciated from overwork or too much exercise, too much heavy lifting, too much sexual activity or if you suffer from chronic vata disorders. It does not need to be accompanied by any strict dietary restriction or daily routine and can be administered, in appropriate cases, at all times of the year. It gives strength, promotes weight gain and helps elimination of waste products.
- *Karma basti* – a schedule of 30 bastis.
- *Kala basti* – a schedule of 15 bastis; ten oil and five decoction.

- *Yoga basti* is a schedule of 8 bastis; five oil and three decoction.
- Nutritional enema (*Bruhana basti*) is used for providing deep nutrition in select conditions. Traditionally, highly nutritive substances have been used, such as warm milk, meat broth, bone marrow soup and herbs such as shatavari or ashwagandha.

Note: In karma, kala and yoga bastis, it is better if you are given both types of basti – oil and decoction – in combination, rather than as separate enemas. In general, the indications and contraindications that apply to enema therapy also apply here.

Indications for enema therapy

- Constipation
- Low back ache
- Gout
- Rheumatism
- Sciatica
- Arthritis
- Nervous disorders
- Vata headache
- Emaciation
- Muscular atrophy

Contraindications

This list is by no means complete, but enema therapy should definitely not be used if you are suffering from any of the following: diarrhoea, bleeding of the rectum, chronic indigestion, breathlessness, diabetes, fever, emaciation, severe anaemia, pulmonary tuberculosis. It is also unsuitable for the elderly or for children below the age of 7 years.

OTHER CONTRAINDICATIONS
The following contraindications apply in the case of specific types of enema:

- **Oil enemas:** diabetes, obesity, indigestion, low digestive fire (agni), enlarged liver or spleen, unconsciousness, tuberculosis and cough
- **Decoction enemas:** debility, hiccough, haemorrhoids, inflammation of anus, piles, diarrhoea, pregnancy, ascites, diabetes and some conditions involving painful or difficult breathing
- **Nutritional enemas:** diabetes, obesity, lymphatic obstruction, ascites
- **Urethra or vaginal enemas:** diabetes

NASAL THERAPY

In ayurveda, the nose is considered the doorway to the brain and it is also the doorway to consciousness. Nasal administration of medication is called *nasya*. Any excess of bodily doshas accumulated in the sinus, throat, nose or head areas is eliminated by means of the nearest possible opening, the nose.

Life energy or the breath of life (*prana*) – enters the body through the breath taken in through the nose. Prana is centred in the brain and maintains sensory and motor functions. It also governs mental processes, memory, concentration and intellect. Unbalanced or deranged prana creates defective functioning of all these activities and produces headaches, convulsions, memory loss and reduced sensory perception. Thus nasya is indicated for prana disorders, sinus congestion, migraines, convulsions and certain eye and ear problems.

Breathing can also be improved through nasal massage. For this treatment, the practitioner dips his or her little finger into ghee (clarified butter) and gently inserts it into your nose. The inner walls of the nose are slowly massaged, going as deeply as possible without causing pain or damage to the delicate mucus membranes. This treatment will help to open your emotions.

As most people have a deviated nasal septum, one side of your nose will usually be easier to penetrate and massage than the other. The finger should never be inserted forcibly. The massage should proceed slowly, with the practitioner moving his or her finger first in a clockwise and then in a counterclockwise direction. By this means, any emotions blocked in the respiratory tract will be released.

Nasal therapy can be used morning and evening. Your breathing patterns will change as your emotions are released and your eyesight also will improve.

There are six main types of nasal therapy. These are:

- Cleansing nasal therapy (*Pradhamana nasya*) – uses dry powders (rather than oils) that are blown into the nose through a tube. It is mainly used for kapha-type diseases involving headaches, heaviness in the head, colds, nasal congestion, sticky eyes, hoarseness of voice due to sticky kapha, sinusitis, cervical lymph adenitis, tumours, worms, some skin diseases, epilepsy, drowsiness, Parkinson's disease, inflammation of the nasal membranes, attachment, greed and lust. Traditionally, powders such as brahmi are used.

- Nutrition nasal therapy (*Bruhana nasya*) uses ghee, oils, salt, shatavari ghee, ashwagandha ghee and medicated milk. It is used mainly for vata disorders. It is said to benefit conditions resulting from vata imbalances such as vata-type headaches, migraines, dryness of voice, dry nose, nervousness, anxiety, fear, dizziness, emptiness, negativity, heaviness of eyelids, bursitis, stiffness in the neck, dry sinuses and loss of sense of smell.
- Sedative nasal therapy (*Shaman nasya*) is used according to which dosha is aggravated, but mainly for pitta-type disorders such as thinning hair, conjunctivitis and ringing in the ears. Generally, certain herbal medicated decoctions, teas and medicated oils are used.
- Decoction nasal therapy (*Navana nasya*) is used in vata-pitta or kapha-pitta disorders and is made from decoctions and oils combined.
- Ghee or oil nasal therapy (*Marshya nasya*).
- Daily oil nasla therapy (*Prati marshya*) is performed by dipping the clean little finger in ghee or oil, inserting it into each nostril, and lubricating the nasal passage with gentle massage as described above. This helps to open deep tissues and can be done every day and at any time to relieve stress.

Substances used: Black pepper, brahmi, curry pepper, ginger, ghee, oils, decoctions, onion, garlic, jasmine, rose, mogra flowers and henna.

Indications for nasal therapy

- Stress
- Emotional imbalances
- Stiffness in the neck and shoulders
- Dryness of the nose
- Sinus congestion
- Hoarseness
- Migraine
- Convulsions

Contraindications

- Sinus infections
- Pregnancy
- Menstruation
- Following sex, bathing, eating or drinking alcohol
- Children aged less than 7 years or people over 80 years of age

RAKTAMOKSHA

Toxins present in the gastrointestinal tract are absorbed into the blood and circulated throughout the body. This condition is called toxaemia, and is the basic cause of repeated infections, hypertension and recurring attacks of skin disorders such as urticaria, rashes, herpes, eczema, acne, scabies, leukoderma, chronic itching and hives. With such conditions as these, along with internal medication, the elimination of toxins and purification of the blood is necessary. This treatment is known as *raktamoksha*. It is also used in cases of enlarged liver or spleen, and gout.

Pitta is produced from disintegrated red blood cells in the liver. Hence pitta and blood have a very close relationship. An increase in pitta may spread to the blood, causing toxicity and many other pitta-type disorders. Extracting a small amount of blood from a vein relieves the tension created by pittagenic toxins in the blood. Bloodletting also stimulates the spleen to produce antitoxic substances that help to boost the immune system. Toxins are neutralized, enabling radical cures in many blood-borne disorders.

Bloodletting is contraindicated in cases of anaemia, oedema, extreme weakness, diabetes and in children and elderly people. It is an illegal procedure in the USA.

Certain substances such as sugar, salt, yogurt, sour-tasting foods and alcohol are toxic to the blood. In some blood disorders, these substances should be avoided to keep the blood pure. Burdock-root tea, sandalwood, saffron, manjista (*Rubia cordifolia Linn.*), guduchi, rose and lotus are herbs that help to purify the blood. Turmeric, golden seal, neem, oranges, pomegranate juice, beets and raisins can also be beneficial for blood disorders.

For raktamoksha treatment other than bloodletting, there are blood-purifying practices involving herbs, gem therapy (see page 90) and colour water therapy.

For blood-purification therapy, bitter and astringent substances with blood-thinning properties are used. Burdock-root tea is the best blood purifier. For blood-related disorders such as allergy, rash or acne, you should take a milk laxative and, the next evening, begin burdock-root tea therapy. The tea is made from one teaspoon of powder in a cup of hot water. If taken every night, the herbs will begin to purify the blood.

For any raktamoksha treatment or related alternative treatment, it is beneficial to refrain from yogurt, salt, sugar, alcohol, sour and fermented foods.

Indications for raktamoksha

- Urticaria
- Rash
- Acne
- Eczema
- Scabies
- Leukoderma
- Chronic itching
- Hives
- Enlarged liver or spleen
- Gout

Contraindications

- Anaemia
- Oedema
- Weakness
- Young children and the elderly
- Pregnancy
- Menstruation

Advice for care during and after panchakarma

During any step of panchakarma, certain lifestyle and dietary guidelines are recommended. You are advised to get plenty of rest during panchakarma and to avoid strenuous exercise, sexual activity, late nights, loud music, television viewing and other stimulating experiences. You are also advised to take particular care to keep warm and away from the draughts and wind and to observe your thoughts and experiences during this time.

A mono-diet of kitchari (a seasoned mixture of rice and moong dal, see page 101) and ghee (clarified butter) is recommended). You should restrict your intake of cold drinks, cold food, caffeine, white sugar, recreational drugs, alcohol and dairy products. These substances should not be resumed (if at all) until some time after panchakarma is completed. This diet is necessary because your digestive fire (agni) takes a rest during the cleansing process. Also, as toxins move back into the gastrointestinal tract, the power of digestion is further slowed. Kitchari is basic to the ayurvedic way of life. It nourishes all the tissues of the body, is very easy to digest, is excellent for the rejuvenation of cells and assists in the detoxification and cleansing process. Basmati rice and moong dal both have the

qualities of being sweet and cooling with a sweet aftertaste. Together, they create a balanced food that is an excellent protein combination and is suitable for all three doshas and therefore any constitution.

Note: Panchakarma is a very specialist ayurvedic procedure, requiring proper guidance from a highly trained and skilled ayurvedic doctor with a minimum of a university degree and five years' experience. It is individually tailored for each person, with their unique constitution and specific disorder in mind, thus it requires close observation and supervision. It is carried out to best advantage, although not always, at the cusp of two seasons, thus helping a person to release accumulated toxins and prepare their internal environment for the forthcoming season.

below **REST, RELAXATION AND A STRESS-FREE ENVIRONMENT ARE IMPORTANT WHEN YOU ARE UNDERGOING PANCHAKARMA**

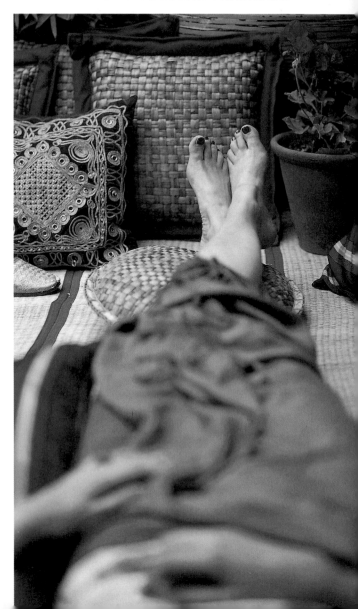

Ayurvedic medicine

Ayurvedic therapy aims to treat and cure the patient of any acute, chronic or underlying physical disease or imbalance in the doshas. There are ayurvedic medicines available that help restore equilibrium between the three doshas. Usually, these medicines are a mixture of plant and herbal extracts and are prepared under suitable pharmaceutical and manufacturing conditions. Minerals and metals are also sometimes used. They are available in several forms.

Asava and arista – A fermented product prepared by placing the required drug extracts in solution for a specified period of time. During this period, a biochemical process of fermentation occurs. The fermentation produces alcohol (which also serves as a preservative) and allows the active principles from the drug extracts to be drawn out. There are several asavas and aristas manufactured in ayurveda, such as abhayarishtam, balarishtam and lohasavam.

Avaleha or lehya – These are semi-solid preparations created by using a decoction of the drugs and adding either sugar or jaggery (palm sugar) to the mixture, which is then boiled and ready for use. Some of the most commonly used medicines are agastya haritaki rasayana and kutajavaleha.

Bhasma – This involves calcination of the drug extracts to yield a powdered dosage formulation. The main ingredients for bhasmas come from animals, minerals and metals, which undergo burning and are reduced to ash. For example, the conch shell is used to make sankha bhasma.

Choornam – For this form of medicine, the drug ingredients are dried thoroughly and pounded using a mortar and pestle to produce a finely or coarsely powdered form of the drugs. Choornams such as vacha choornam, amrutha choornam and avipathi choornam are used for ayurvedic treatment.

Ghrta – Ghee (clarified butter) is the main ingredient, and drug extracts are added to it and boiled with it. By following this procedure, the drug's active ingredients become absorbed in the ghee and thus generate ayurvedic medicines, such as dasamoola ghrta and triphala ghrta.

Guggulu – These are preparations where the extract from the plant *Commifora mukul* is the main active ingredient in the medicine. There are various types of guggulu used today, such as kancanara guggulu, kaisora guggulu and vyosadi guggulu.

Hima – A cold infusion, hima is generated by mixing one part of the extract with eight parts water, which is then left overnight. Thereafter, the mixture is filtered through a fine muslin cloth before use.

Kashayam or kwatha – These are coarsely powdered drugs that are placed into a vessel containing four, eight or sixteen parts water. They are then vigorously boiled to reduce them to a quarter of their original volume, filtered and the decoction separated. A large proportion of the medicines used today are kashayams; these include dhanwantharam kashayam, indukantha kashayam and rasnadi kashayam.

Lepa – The drug extracts are ground into a fine powder, then a paste is subsequently produced by adding a little water or another liquid. This form of ayurvedic medicine is for external use only. Dasanga lepa, pathyadi lepa and sothanghna lepa are a few examples.

Swarasa or rasa – This is a liquid formulation produced by pounding the appropriate drug in its fresh plant form to obtain its juice, which is then strained through a clean cloth. There are many rasayanams, including agastya rasayanam, narsimha rasayanam and dasamoola rasayanam.

Taila – There are several steps in the synthesis of oils, or tailas. The oil is the main ingredient to which drugs are added, and the resulting mixture is then boiled. The active ingredients from the drug extracts are absorbed into the oil. The method of preparation for ghees and tailas is very similar. There are several ayurvedic oils used today, such as anu taila, hingu triguna taila and ksheerabala taila. These oils are generally for external use.

Vatika and gutika – These are tablets or pills made up from one or more ingredients. The active ingredients mainly come from vegetables, minerals and metals. This is a very convenient form of medicine to take, coming as it does in measured doses, and is more suitable for certain patients than other treatments. Khadira gutika, eladi gutika and gandhaka vati are some of the tablets used in ayurvedic treatment.

Under the holistic principles of ayurveda, all plants and other resources used in ayurvedic medicine must be grown, cultivated, collected and stored under appropriate conditions and with due consideration for the environment. The medicines are also available in different types of ayurvedic formulations, because certain people will prefer one particular dosage form to another. They also provide the same medicines in a choice of preparations.

Shirodhara

Shirodhara is a healing therapy unique to ayurveda. It was initially conceived and practised by ayurvedic healers in Kerala, India. Hence the details of this therapy are found in the ayurvedic literature of Kerala. According to the experts, it is very effective in treating mental illnesses such as depression, anxiety, mania and psychosis. However, the ancient texts tell us that it can be used even for physical diseases such as hair loss, insomnia, heart disease and headache as well. Recent studies also show that it is very effective in treating hypertension (high blood pressure).

Shiras means 'head', while *dhara* means 'stream'. Usually, when you are having this treatment, a thin stream of warm oil is allowed to flow slowly and continuously over your forehead and head, hence its name of shirodhara. Other liquids such as buttermilk (processed with gooseberry), milk, breast milk and plain water may also be used.

All the nerves of your body meet at a point on your forehead between your eyebrows, known as the 'third eye'. The stream of oil seems first to affect the qualities of mind, the gunas of satvic, rajas and tamas, which in turn affect the physical doshas of vata, pitta and kapha. The slow, continuous, soothing flow of oil or buttermilk over a period of 30 to 45 minutes helps you to relax completely, making it very useful in treating any stress-related condition. One of the main advantages of this therapy is that it does not require an elaborate set-up or expensive technology, or a stay in a resort or hospital. It can be administered effectively on an outpatient basis. As is the case with all ayurvedic treatment, it should only be carried out by a skilled, qualified practitioner.

Materials required

- A treatment table, 1.8–2 m (6½–7 ft) long, 0.75–1 m (2½–3ft) wide, preferably wooden
- A dhara pot, earthen or metallic, with a hole in the centre about the size of a little finger
- A stand from which to hang the dhara pot
- Dhara medicine – oil or buttermilk, for example
- Cotton thread to prepare the wick
- Bowls to collect the oil
- Cotton pads

How is it done?

- Before the treatment itself begins, you will be asked to empty your bowels and bladder.
- You will then lie down on the table, face up.

- A gentle head massage is then given which will help you to relax before the actual treatment starts.
- Next, your eyes will be covered with cotton pads soaked in cold milk and your ears plugged with cotton swabs.
- The dhara pot will then be adjusted over your forehead, with the dhara wick approximately four fingers in width above your forehead.
- The oil or buttermilk is then poured into the dhara pot and allowed to flow steadily and comfortably over your forehead in a relaxing stream. The oil must be lukewarm. (If buttermilk is used, there is no need for warming – however, it will be at room temperature.)
- The dhara pot is rotated or oscillated in such a way that the oil or buttermilk gently and rhythmically flows over your entire forehead in a soothing manner.
- You will then be asked to relax, breathe deeply and meditate.
- The oil flows from your head to be collected in bowls placed beneath the treatment table, and is periodically returned to the dhara pot to ensure the flow of oil is continuous.
- This part of the procedure will take place for about 45 minutes to one hour. There must be absolute silence in the therapy room throughout.
- After the allotted time, you will be asked to sit up slowly and your forehead and head will be cleaned with a towel.

Shirodhara is best carried out on an empty stomach, so avoid having it directly after meals. You should shower one to two hours after the treatment and then follow a light diet, eating only when you feel hungry. The procedure may be carried out for one, two or three weeks at a stretch, and it is advisable to avoid heavy, stressful activities during this period. A cup of milk boiled with powdered ginger and sugar candy may be prescribed to you while you are undergoing shirodhara. You should also wash your hair with rasnadi choornam.

What are its benefits?

- Shirodhara is relaxing and helps you to overcome daily stresses and strains
- Useful for insomnia and headaches
- Good for patients suffering from mental illnesses such as depression, anxiety neurosis, psychosis and mania
- Reduces blood pressure in hypertensive patients
- Good for hair loss, baldness and greying hair

right THE RELAXING ART OF SHIRODHARA IS BENEFICIAL IN TREATING AILMENTS SUCH AS MIGRAINE, ANXIETY AND INSOMNIA

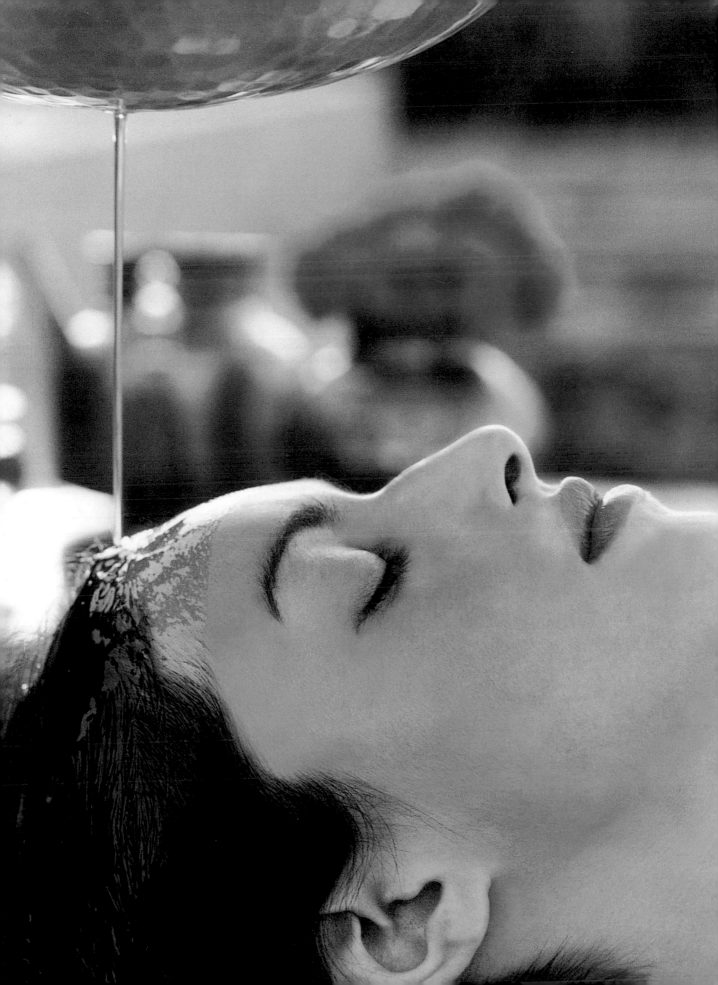

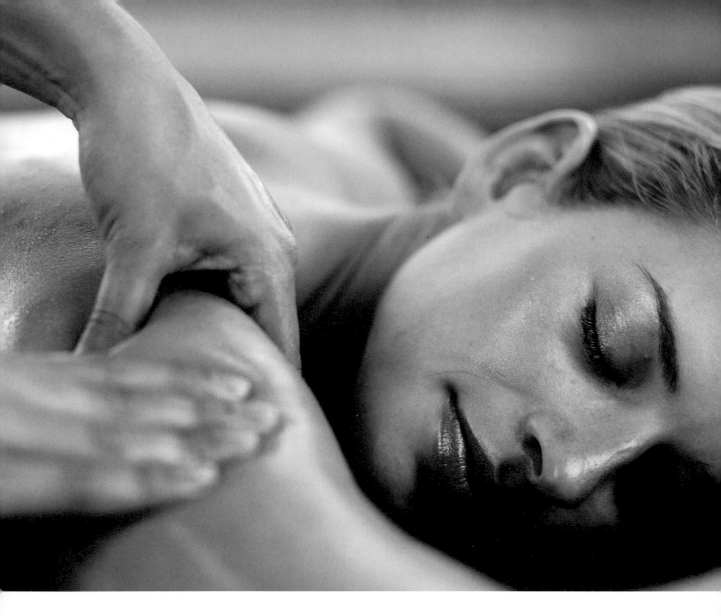

Ayurvedic massage

In ayurveda, massage is highly recommended as a part of your daily routine. It is also recommended as a therapy either independently or as preparation for treatment by panchakarma.

Ayurveda views aches and pains as the result of the obstruction of the flow of air (*vayu*). Massage performed with particular oils helps to release the obstruction and free the movement of vayu, thereby resulting in relief from any physical discomfort.

Massage is given through the sense of touch. The skin is the largest organ in the body and the main seat of vata, as well as a vehicle for tactile sensations. A balanced and unobstructed vata is necessary for the proper relay of these sensations. Ayurvedic massage is able to provide this, as it helps your body's energy to flow while at the same time releasing toxins.

Benefits of ayurvedic massage

- Reduces the effects of ageing
- Removes fatigue
- Removes excess wind
- Improves vision
- Strengthens the body
- Increases longevity
- Induces sleep and dreams
- Strengthens the skin
- Aids resistance to disharmony and disease
- Soothes ailments caused by wind and mucus
- Improves the colour and texture of the skin

above and right **MASSAGE CAN HAVE MANY BENEFITS FOR YOUR HEALTH. REGULAR OIL MASSAGES AND A DRY MASSAGE AT THE CHANGE OF SEASONS IS RECOMMENDED FOR MOST PEOPLE. YOU CAN EVEN MAKE IT PART OF YOUR DAILY ROUTINE**

Massage nourishes all the seven tissues – plasma, blood, muscle, fat, bone, nerves and reproductive – balances the three doshas, rejuvenates your system, increases strength and vitality, cures disease and removes stress and strain.

In ayurveda, there are three forms of oil massage:

- Abyhanga – full body massage
- Pizzhichil – usually given by four masseurs with oil poured on the body continuously throughout
- Chavutti thirumal – using a combination of poured oil and the masseur's feet

Ayurvedic head and foot massage

Although it is best to have your entire body massaged, this is a time-consuming process. If time is short, try to massage at least your head, feet and ears each day.

Choose the oil most suitable for your prakruti (see right), and gently warm it before use. Sit on a low stool or a towel on the floor, making sure that the spot you choose is free from draughts. Apply the oil to the appropriate part of your body and allow it to absorb for a few minutes. Next, using a combination of gentle, circular movements with your fingertips, and up-and-down strokes with the heel of your hand, smooth the oil into your skin. Repeat each movement three times.

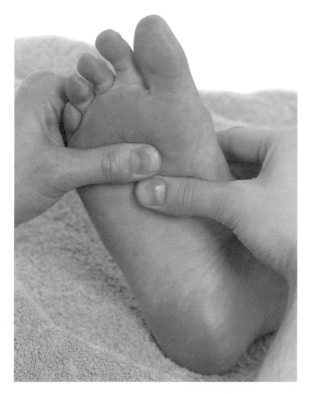

Oils for massage

Ayurveda emphasizes the correct use of different oils in massage. They should be used according to the seasons and the particular requirements of your body. In fact, ayurvedic practice places more emphasis on using specific oils for specific body type or dosha imbalances than it does on techniques. The oils should be selected on the basis of their effect on the doshas. For example:

- Vata – sesame oil
- Pitta – coconut oil
- Kapha – mustard oil or olive oil

There are hundreds of processed herbal medicinal oils available in ayurveda. They can also be selected on the basis of their effect on dosha and on particular disease types. For example:

- Vata/vata diseases – Dhanwantaram tailam
  Bala tailam
  Sahacharadi tailam

- Pitta/pitta diseases – Chandanadi tailam
  ,
  Ksheerabala tailam

- Kapha/kapha diseases – Triphala tailam
  Asana bilwadi tailam
  Tulasyadi tailam

Sometimes, particular oils are used specifically for certain conditions. For example:

- Joint pain/arthritis – Sahacharadi tailam
  Dhanwantaram tailam

- Insomnia – Himasagara tailam

- Anxiety/mania – Chandanadi tailam

- Headache – Asana bilwadi tailam

A cautionary note

Although massage is generally beneficial to your health and wellbeing, and has some curative properties, it should not be used in the following circumstances: when you are suffering from ama (toxins) or kapha imbalances, or if you are very obese, pregnant, suffering from a skin disease or following a heavy meal.

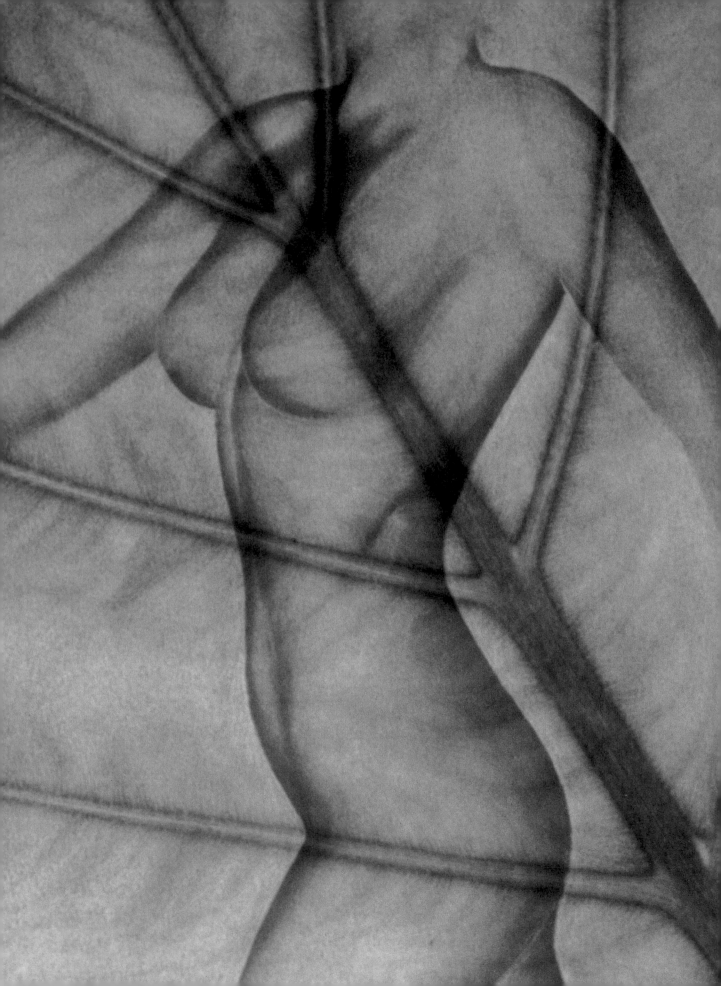

4 ayurveda and allied therapies

Ayurveda for a healthy lifestyle

Health is the first prerequisite of all attainments in life. The attainment of health is not only an individual human aspiration, but also a basic human right.

World Health Organization

Medicine, almost more than any other human activity, touches every home. Today, many health problems, particularly chronic ones, are not amenable to treatment by conventional medical technologies, which can be expensive, have undesirable side effects or are of doubtful effectiveness. The ayurvedic approach to health and wellbeing often provides a better alternative. Ayurveda has simple, inexpensive and time-tested treatment regimes and remedies which are easily accessible to people in any society. Its acceptance and validity rest on a long tradition of practice over more than 5,000 years, and it has at its heart the following aims and objectives.

- Prevention, preservation and promotion of health and mental wellbeing
- Promotion of an ideal constitution
- Healthy living through improving the quality of your body's tissues and your quality and strength of mind
- Effective treatment of disease

In ayurveda, a natural approach to health promotion and disease prevention is practised. With traditional Western medicine, only a specific group of diseases can be prevented, and treatment of disease usually

left **HEALTH IS THE FOUNDATION UPON WHICH OUR HAPPINESS DEPENDS. DAILY ROUTINE IS A KEY PART OF ACHIEVING THIS**

focusses on the disease only and not the body as a whole. Also, the natural ability of your body to adapt itself and face new illnesses or a recurrence of the original disease is often almost eliminated by these measures. Ayurveda advocates the following natural preventive measures:

- Daily routine (*dinacharya*)
- Seasonal routine (*ritucharya*)

Together, these regimes are known as *swashtavritta*, the conduct of healthy living.

Daily routine

If your aim is a long, healthy life, you must keep yourself healthy from day to day. Ayurveda's daily routine, which includes care of the body, mind and sense organs, helps you do this. Exercise, sex, sleep, personal hygiene, religious practices and other daily activities are an aspect of this. These activities influence each organ and your body as a whole, helping you to achieve perfect physical and mental health, and maintaining the normal biorhythms of your body, another important aspect of wellbeing.

- The ideal time for waking is before sunrise. Start your day with prayer and meditation, and focus on auspicious objects for a pleasant and successful day. Take the time to plan your actions.
- Empty your bowels and bladder immediately after this, so that you develop regular bowel habits. This also helps to evacuate any metabolic wastes accumulated in your body overnight. Drinking a glass of tepid water when you first wake can encourage regularity.
- Caring for your mouth, teeth and tongue is the next crucial step. Washing your face with herbal decoctions, cleaning your teeth with herbal

powder or toothpaste, and regularly scraping your tongue with a metallic or wooden tongue-scraper should be part of your daily routine. Herbal gargles also have a place in your daily routine, as they help to enhance your sense of taste. They also improve your voice, complexion and sense of smell.

• Looking after your various sense organs – eyes, ears, nose and skin – is also very important.

Looking after your eyes – Eye ointment should be regularly applied using a proper applicator. Triphala decoction helps maintain your eyes' health.

Looking after your ears – Sesame oil or coconut oil drops should be instilled in the ears daily.

Nasal care – Two drops of medicated oil (*anu taila*) should be routinely instilled in each nostril.

Skincare – Massaging the body with sesame oil helps to improve your skin's complexion and your hair's lustre. It also tones muscles and blood vessels, and soothes your skin and nervous system. Your head, ears and the soles of your feet, particularly, should be massaged regularly (see pages 66–7). Herbal powders and pastes can also be rubbed into the skin to improve the complexion.

In addition to these measures, mental and moral discipline is an aspect of your daily routine that should not be overlooked. In keeping with ayurveda's holistic nature, your mental health and wellbeing are just as vital as your physical health. You should try to avoid negative feelings, such as greed, vanity, jealousy and anger, and avoid people who display these attributes as part of their basic nature. It is also important to show respect for others and to help them out in times of difficulty. Be decisive, fearless and forgiving, and make good use of your intelligence.

Seasonal routines

The existence and wellbeing of humans and other living organisms depend on the continuous interaction and adjustment between their external and internal environment. These factors are continuously changing according to the seasons. In order to adjust to seasonal changes, you need to change your living pattern, clothing and food habits accordingly. The seasonal routine describes the influence of various seasons on the human body and the necessary adjustments you should make to your lifestyle.

There are six seasons according to the Hindu calendar: *Vasantha* (spring), *Greeshma* (summer), *Varsha* (rainy

Looking after your body

The body is believed to be sustained on three pillars of health: nutrition, sleep and sex, and spirituality. You should therefore use them judiciously to maintain your physical health.

• Take regular exercise. Regular, systematic exercise is necessary to increase your body's strength and stability. Exercising before you eat breakfast is good for your circulation and keeping your doshas in balance, while a short, brisk walk after breakfast will aid your digestion. Again, as with all things, moderation is important. Too much or even inappropriate exercise can be as damaging to your health as too little.

• Regular baths should be taken, either with hot or cold water, or with medicated decoctions.

• You should always wear clean, soft clothes. They should be appropriate to your personality and protect your body, and you should change your clothing according to the season. A cap or hat to protect your head, as well as an umbrella for rainy weather and suitable footwear to protect your feet, are also vital whenever you are travelling. Perfume, cosmetics and jewellery that suit your personality and culture may be worn.

• You must make sure that your diet is moderate, well balanced and nutritious. Your intake should be moderate, with plenty of fresh foods, and also take into account your digestive capacity (agni).

• Make sure that you get six to eight hours sleep every night; sleeping during the day, however, should be avoided.

• The sexual drive is primary to all human beings, but you should exercise suitable control over this instinct and not indulge it to excess. Moderation in sexual activity is recommended and you should never practice sexual behaviour that is harmful to you or to others.

• Natural urges (autonomic reflexes) such as hunger, thirst, urination, sleep and sneezing should not be withheld or suppressed, nor should they be induced unnecessarily. This does not mean you should give into harmful psychological urges such as greed, fear, anger and vanity.

In short, controlled and conscious exercise of the body and mind is essential for maintaining sound health. The daily routine is aimed at achieving this goal. This protocol should be adopted after taking into consideration your age, sex, strength, prakruti, mental health, agni, external environment and any disease from which you are suffering. Once again, the aim is holistic: mental and physical wellbeing.

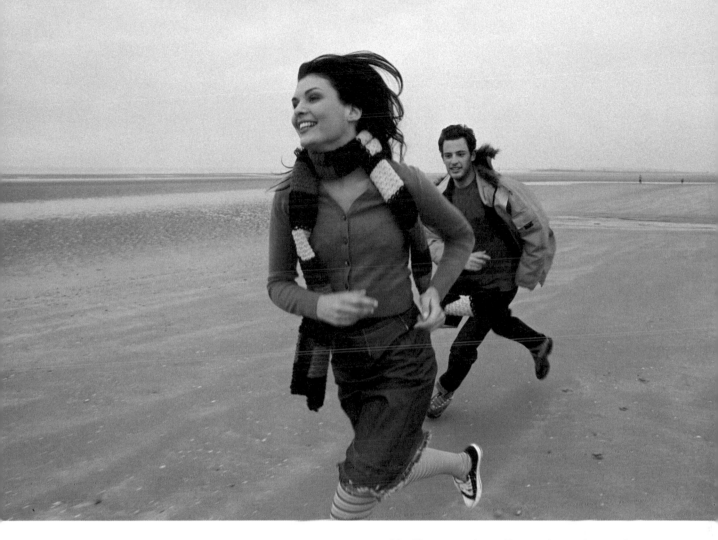

above **LOOKING AFTER YOUR BODY IS AN IMPORTANT PRINCIPLE IN AYURVEDA. MAKE SURE YOU GET REGULAR EXERCISE AND ALWAYS DRESS APPROPRIATELY FOR THE SEASON**

season), *Sarath* (autumn), *Hemantha* (the cold period before winter) and *Shishira* (winter). In most Western countries, these translate to three seasons according to ayurvedic principles: kapha season (spring to early summer), pitta season (summer to mid-autumn) and vata season (mid-autumn to early spring).

The need to prepare your body and mind for each season is why it is recommended that you undergo panchakarma, or cleansing therapy, at the change of the seasons (see pages 54–61). You should also bear in mind that, when a season matches your prakruti, or body type, you will need to be especially careful about aggravating that particular dosha. For instance, vata-type problems are more likely during the vata season, so you should take account of this if vata is your dominant dosha. Another aspect of the seasonal routine relating to your prakruti is temperature. If you have a vata constitution, you need to avoid excessive cold, wind, rain and snow during winter. Wrap up well and avoid exposure to the elements as much as

possible. Pitta types do not like very hot or dry weather, and so should avoid the sun as much as possible in the heat of summer and make sure that they are always adequately hydrated. If kapha dominates your prakruti, you will be uncomfortable in humid and cold climates.

While it is important that each of us consider our prakruti with regard to each season, there are some general guidelines about diet and lifestyle which apply universally and relate to the dominant dosha of the season. You should follow a warm, nourishing diet in winter. Favour cooked foods and warm drinks, and dress to ensure protection against the cold. In summer, you will need to follow a diet which does not aggravate pitta and has a cooling effect. Drink plenty of cool water and avoid taking hot baths.

Foods for vata season – almonds, buttermilk, eggs, fish, ghee (clarified butter), green beans, oats.

Foods for pitta season – apples, avocado, butter, chicken, chickpeas, eggs, fish, rice, spinach, wheat.

Foods for kapha season – apricots, broccoli, chicken, chillies, fish, garlic, okra, onion, rice, spinach, tomato.

Ensuring an ideal constitution

Every individual has a unique constitution or prakruti (see pages 28–35). The responses, durability and resistance of the seven body tissues depend on your individual prakruti. As your prakruti and the qualities of body tissues are fixed at birth, you must try to make sure that any children you have will be as healthy and strong as possible. In ayurveda, the following guidelines are given for making certain you have a healthy pregnancy and that there is a safe, successful outcome for your baby:

- Marriage should take place at the right age so that the couples can reproduce during the right period. A child born to an older couple or to a very young couple will be genetically weak. A close blood relationship should be avoided.
- Women should follow rules and regulations suggested in ayurveda during their menstrual period. These include: no heavy exertion, no sex and avoiding situations that make you anxious.
- Certain regimes, rituals and rules must be followed for lovemaking to ensure a genetically strong child.
- Antenatal, natal and postnatal care, as prescribed in ayurveda, should be followed.

If a child is born with a weak constitution and poor resistance, ayurveda advises rejuvenation therapy (see page 86) to improve tissue resistance. This will help to combat early degeneration and deterioration.

A strong and healthy mind

The human mind has some very mysterious powers. It can convert an enemy into a friend, a moment into years, hell into heaven and a man into a god. The mind controls all the activities of the body. Mental health is a primary requisite for happiness and longevity.

In ayurvedic practice, your personal and social conduct (sadvritta) has a great bearing on your mental health and wellbeing, and strict mental discipline and a strong moral base are considered crucial. Yoga is another discipline that is aimed at achieving perfect mental health (see pages 82–3). The following basic tenets for personal and social conduct should be adopted and stand at the core of your behaviour and attitude.

- Follow and respect the rules of your religion
- Do not take part in activities unthinkingly. Always consider and take note of your actions and their consequences

- Never be inactive or idle. This does not mean that you should never relax, but rather that you should not let time slip by without conscious thought
- Perform your duty at the right time and in the right manner
- Develop a detached attitude
- Fulfil your duty without any expectation of reward
- Be socially responsible
- Respect your elders, serving the poor and the aged

Sleep, rest and relaxation

According to the *Charaka Samhita*, happiness, misery, nourishment, emaciation, strength, weakness, virility, sterility, knowledge, ignorance, life and death, are all dependent upon proper or improper sleep patterns. Sleep serves an very important restorative function; its purpose is similar to that of diet in providing nourishment. Sleep gives the mind a chance to rest.

One of the most important aspects of your lifestyle is to maintain a proper balance in the rest and activity cycle. Of all the rhythmical cycles that constitute the progression of time, none is more important than the sleep–wake system. Unfortunately, the sleep–wake system is also the most neglected. Ninety per cent of people in modern industrialized societies suffer from chronic sleep deficit – a condition that is known to cause increased susceptibility to infectious diseases, increased incidence of gastrointestinal disorders and cardiovascular disease. It also influences our mood.

Too little sleep or irregular sleep patterns will cause an aggravation of vata. Aggravated vata also causes the other two doshas to become unbalanced. Therefore, in order to keep our doshas in balance and enjoy health and happiness, good sleep is necessary.

The sleep–wake system is inextricably linked to lifestyle and to your mental, physical and emotional condition. The intake of recreational drugs, some types of medication, alcohol and smoking are all known to be associated with sleep disorders. So are an erratic and irregular lifestyle and poor eating habits, especially eating heavily in the evening. Long-term sleep disorders indicate deeper imbalances in the vata and pitta doshas, whereas too much sleep during the daytime unbalances kapha.

The ayurvedic prescription for a good night's sleep is:

- Relax with an oil massage
- Maintain a tranquil and serene state of mind
- Create a restful atmosphere in your bedroom
- Do not work or watch television in the bedroom

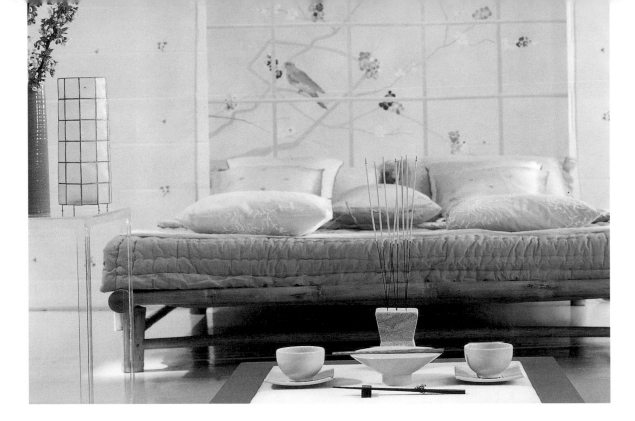

above **YOUR BEDROOM SHOULD BE A PEACEFUL OASIS OF REST AND RELAXATION. IT IS NOT A GOOD IDEA TO COMBINE IT WITH A HOME OFFICE OR WATCH TELEVISION THERE. BURNING INCENSE IS NOT RECOMMENDED FOR ANYONE WITH RESPIRATORY PROBLEMS**

- Be involved in a good, supportive relationship
- Refrain from drugs, smoking, alcohol, caffeine and sleeping pills
- Make sure you have healthy eating habits. Avoid heavy meals, especially in the evening, and do not eat too late in the evening
- Indulge in soothing baths
- Take regular exercise
- Drink a cup of hot or warm milk at bedtime
- Practice yoga and meditation

Balanced behaviour

According to Charaka, the overuse or misuse of any one of the five senses can also have serious effects on our health. Our behaviour is our reaction to the knowledge and experience derived from our sense organs as well as our minds. For instance, Charaka states that misuse of sight is to 'see things that are awful or terrifying, frightful, deformed or alarming'.

The health effects of behaviour are poorly understood and little studied in modern medicine. We know that we get material for the reconstruction of our bodies through the food we eat. On a more subtle level, we also get it through the energy we take in mentally and emotionally. The 'drama of life' as it is played out on the screen of our mind is 'metabolized' and transformed into physiological reality according to Maharishi Mahesh Yogi. Every thought, emotion and experience is associated with a unique pattern of neuronal and biochemical activity. Neuro-endocrinology has recently arrived at the understanding that positive emotions evoke physiological processes which support our health and wellbeing, while negative emotions do the reverse. Put simply, laughter is the best medicine.

The key term in ayurveda, with respect to behaviour, is 'moderation'. Too much of any one thing is an overload and will unbalance the doshas. Anger, passion or lust, grief and fear unbalance vata dosha, and anger also upsets pitta. Too much sensual pleasure depletes reproductive tissue, and all emotions in excess lower our immunity and resistance.

Sex and relationships

Daily life is enmeshed in our relationships – both with others and with ourselves. Ideally, clarity, compassion and love should characterize these relationships. It is often easier to love and respect others than to love and respect yourself. Relationships should be used as mirrors, reflecting values, emotions and attitudes to which we aspire and which we desire in our own lives. If relationships are ill-defined and tenuous, confusion and conflict arise, which in turn affect wellbeing.

A relationship that is strained, leading to emotional imbalance, also leads to imbalance in our doshas. Fear and anxiety increases vata, anger and hate upset pitta, while attachment and greed imbalances kapha.

Diet and the doshas

Our daily intake of food constitutes the first of the three pillars of life and is the most crucial. Eating is a fundamental physiological activity that maintains our health on a day-to-day basis. Food constitutes the basic energy source from which is formed not only our body, but the quality of the mind and intellect as well. All aspects of our daily diet – what we eat, how we eat and when we eat – are important.

The ancient ayurvedic text *Charaka Samhita notes* that 'wholesome food is one of the causes for the growth of living beings and unwholesome food for the growth of diseases'. Modern researchers know that five out of ten major causes of death – including heart disease, diabetes and cancer – are diet related. Ninety per cent of patients who seek a doctor's advice do so for problems related to their diet, for example obesity, clogged arteries, allergies and sore joints. Eating the right food in the right quantity is a potent requirement for preventing diseases and extending our life span.

A large proportion of people all over the world suffer from digestion-related problems, such as wind, bloating, stomach pains, constipation, heartburn and fatigue after eating. Ayurvedic medicine provides simple solutions to these common complaints by considering not only what we eat, but also how and when we eat it. For example, how many times have you seen someone munching on a sandwich while driving through traffic? How many times have we eaten at our workstation because we did not have time for a proper lunch?

The act of eating, according to ayurveda, is akin to a sacred ritual, as it is important for the development of our conscious, as well as our physical, health. When we sit down to eat, our stomach should be in a relaxed posture and we should be aware of the taste, texture and smell of the food. This will greatly improve our digestion. Our bodies need an uplifting and settled environment in order to process and absorb the nutrients from our meals. If this is not possible, we should at least be sitting down to eat – not standing, walking or driving our way through a meal.

Balancing your agni (digestive capacity) is a vital principle in ayurvedic medicine. That is why ayurveda recommends a number of general practices for better digestion. Agni can be compared to a burning fire. If the flame is very low, it will take a long time to cook the food. In the same way, if the fire is too strong, it will burn the food. Our digestive fire should be balanced so that we can digest meals efficiently and smoothly.

To improve digestion, it is necessary to stimulate the agni before we begin eating. Weak agni may result in fatigue after eating, so ayurveda recommends eating a piece of fresh ginger with a pinch of salt before a full meal. This activates the salivary glands, producing the enzymes necessary for the body to absorb the food's nutrients efficiently and easily. If, on the other hand, you suffer from overactive agni because there is too much internal heat and acid, then you will find that pomegranate chutney is more suitable.

Ayurveda does not recommend taking cold drinks with meals or ice-cold foods in general. This is like pouring cold water on burning logs. Iced water, often served in restaurants, extinguishes the digestive fire. Even juice or milk straight out of the refrigerator is too cold for digestion. Fruit juice should be drunk at room temperature and water without ice. Once you are in the habit of drinking beverages at room temperature, you will notice a dramatic improvement in your digestion and the way your body feels while you are eating and after a meal. Cold drinks and foods mixed with warm, cooked foods can cause stomach cramps, bloating and general discomfort.

The next recommendation has to do with the time of day at which you eat your meals. Have you ever gone out for a late dinner and found that it was a strain to wake up the next morning or that it was difficult to be efficient the next day? These are the side effects of improperly digested food. The best way to avoid these problems is to follow nature's prescription of suitable times to eat. When the sun is strongest between 12 pm and 2 pm, the digestive fire is also strong. Agni is associated with the sun. This is one of the ways in which ayurveda seeks to connect our mind and body with the environment. The largest meal of the day should be lunch, as this is the time that our agni is working at peak efficiency. As the sun goes down, so does our agni.

Your evening meal should be lighter than lunch, and it should ideally be eaten before 8 pm. Late-night meals interfere with sleep and, after 10 pm, the body is working to burn off toxins and continue to digest food from the day. If you eat after 10 pm, the food may cause toxins to accumulate in your system. As a result, you will wake up tired the next day. If you do not wake up feeling fresh and clear, it is important to analyse how much food you have eaten and when.

Another tip for good digestion is to drink a cup of fresh homemade buttermilk after a meal. Buttermilk is light and contains lactobacilli, necessary bacteria that lubricate the intestines to help digestion proceed smoothly. It also helps to reduce gas and bloating.

Good digestion

- Eat sitting down, in a settled environment. Do not eat in front of the television or with it on in the background, and do not eat 'on the run'.
- Eat a fresh piece of ginger with a little rock salt before a full meal to improve your digestive capacity, or pomegranate chutney to balance pitta if your digestive capacity is overactive.
- Eat breakfast before 8 am and make lunch the biggest meal of the day.
- Drink buttermilk after lunch.
- Avoid ice-cold drinks and food.
- Dinner should be light and eaten before 8 pm. Eating too late upsets your digestive processes.

Eat your greens – every day!

According to ayurveda, dark green, leafy vegetables have an important place in your daily diet – they are considered a particularly nutritious class of vegetable. Modern science, also, says that they contain important minerals such as calcium, magnesium, iron, potassium, vitamin A, vitamin K and vitamins B1 and B2. Dark green, leafy vegetables such as collard greens, spinach, Swiss chard, mustard greens, bok choy, sorrel, turnip greens and many varieties of kale offer rich health benefits. Ayurveda recommends that you have some leafy green vegetables every day to help meet the nutritional requirements for optimal health.

As most of our body consists of water, it is important to keep it properly hydrated. Leafy greens contain nutritious juices that help to replenish liquid and also help to purify the subtle channels of the body known as *srotas*. The natural juices and fibres help to purify and refresh the physiology. They also contain prana, or the breath of life, which provides sustenance to mind and body when we consume greens on a regular basis.

Leafy green vegetables help to balance pitta and kapha. People who need to balance vata should also eat leafy greens, but prepared with ghee or olive oil and spices that balance vata. They are very beneficial for people suffering from skin problems, as they are cooling, gentle, purifying and nourishing for the skin. Due to the high content of calcium and vitamin A, they are highly beneficial for reproductive health and during menopause. They also contain antioxidants that help to prevent ageing and disease.

Some leafy greens are tender and cook very quickly; others, such as kale, may need cooking for longer.

It is best to keep the leaf whole when cooking. If there are tough stems, such as on collard greens and kale, slice the stem into bite-size pieces. These should be cooked until tender or they may cause abdominal discomfort. Buy organic greens whenever possible and choose fresh, moist leaves for the best flavour.

Tastes for balanced nutrition

Ayurvedic medicine describes six rasas, or types of taste (see pages 36–9). The six tastes should also be balanced in the diet for optimum health and nutrition. People who need to balance pitta and kapha generally need to eat more bitter and astringent foods. Ayurvedic spice mixes are convenient ways to incorporate these tastes in your diet.

Most people's diet, particularly in the West, tends to be predominantly of sweet and sour tastes. The sweet taste includes wheat products such as bread, cereal and pasta, rice, milk, ice cream and desserts. The sour taste includes food made from tomato products, such as ketchup, spicy Mexican sauce and pasta sauce, cheese, and citrus fruits and drinks. Too much of these tastes increases heat in the body. Sour foods should be reduced in quantity or preferably avoided by anyone suffering from hyperacidity, hypertension or other signs of pitta imbalance.

It is necessary to include some bitter and astringent tastes in your diet. Internally, the bitter taste helps to balance pitta and kapha. It decreases water retention and is used as a tonic for a congested liver. It is cleansing and helps to take away burning and itching sensations. In excess, it can aggravate vata and dehydrate the body. The astringent taste purifies the blood and helps to balance pitta and kapha. In excess, however, it creates gas and constipation.

BITTER AND ASTRINGENT TASTES
Bitter taste – aloe vera, barley, basil, bitter melon and gourd, fenugreek seeds, Japanese eggplant, leafy greens, lettuce, nettle, rhubarb, turmeric.

Astringent taste – apple, bananas (unripe), chickpeas, green peas, legumes, lentils, pear, pomegranate, raspberries, sprouts, quinoa, tofu.

A convenient way to incorporate the bitter taste into your daily diet is to add fenugreek seeds to your food while cooking, as is done in Indian cuisine. Spices are a quick, convenient and aromatic way of incorporating the more unusual bitter and astringent tastes into your daily diet. With a little effort and creativity, you can get those tastes from many other foods as well.

Menus and recipes

Based on your individual prakruti, the season and time of day, and planned according to the six tastes as explained on page 36), you can tailor-make personal menu options that will keep your doshas balanced at all times. A few sample menus have been suggested below and opposite for easy reference.

Note: The foods given in the suggested menus on these pages are annotated as follows:

G – Grains, breads, cereals, rice and pasta
V – Vegetables and fruits
M – Meat and meat alternatives
D – Dairy, milk and milk products
O – Other foods, sweets, condiments and beverages

right HERBAL TEAS, SUCH AS CAMOMILE, CUMIN, GINGER AND MINT, ARE GOOD DIGESTIVE AIDS. TRY MAKING YOUR OWN BY STEEPING THE HERB IN A GLASS OF HOT WATER. SPECIAL TEAS SUITABLE FOR VATA, PITTA AND KAPHA ARE ALSO AVAILABLE

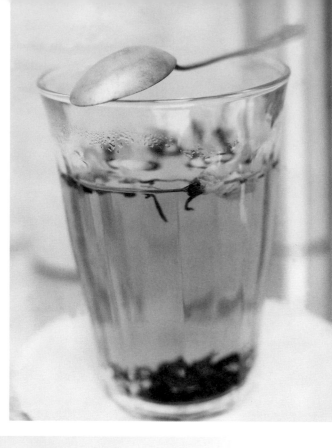

Ideal menu for vata

Breakfast	Oatmeal muffins or pancakes (G)	Creamed wheat porridge (G)
	Seasonal sweet fruits eaten 1 hour before any other food (V)	Milk for porridge, if desired (D)
	Tea with sweetener, if desired	Tea with sweetener, if desired
Lunch	Chapati (G)	Chapati/puri/plain rice (with soup) (G)
	Saffron rice (G)	Cooked carrots sprinkled with fresh lemon juice (V)
	Mixed vegetables (V) or moong dal kitchari (vata) with ghee and coriander (M)	Moong dal kitchari or toor dal soup (M)
	Fresh lemon peanut chutney (O)	Handful of almonds
	Sweet lassi or tea (D)	Fresh lemon (squeeze over the vegetables) (O)
	Tea (have tea 1 hour after lassi)	Sesame chutney (O)
		Vata tea (O)
Snacks	Oatmeal muffins or pancakes (G)	Ginger snaps or sesame snaps (G)
	Seasonal fruits (V)	Seasonal sweet fruit (V)
	Soaked, peeled almonds (M)	Hot spiced milk, especially good before bed (do not have this if you have eaten an egg) (D)
	Hot spiced milk before bed (optional) (D)	Herbal teas or grain coffee with milk (O)
	Herbal teas such as camomile or cumin (O)	
Dinner	Cooked spinach (V)	Chapati (G)
	Tapioca kitchari (M)	Wheat tortilla (G)
	(Note: grains should not be eaten with tapioca kitchari) (G)	Baked sweet potato (V) with an egg or roasted ground sunflower seeds (sprinkle over the potato) (M)
	Fresh lemon or lime for the kitchari (O)	Fresh lemon (O)
	Sweet potato pudding (O)	
	Tea (O)	

Ideal menu for pitta

Breakfast
Oat bran muffin with ghee (clarified butter)
  or oat or wheat granola (G)
Seasonal fruit – eat 1 hour before other food (V)
Milk for cereal, if desired (D)
Mint tea or agni tea (O)

Creamed wheat porridge or oatmeal (G)
Milk or ghee with porridge, if desired (D)
Tea with maple syrup or sweetener (O)

Lunch
Chapati (G)
Boiled basmati rice (G)
Bitter melon or green bean vegetable,
  small salad with oil dressing (V)
Pachak lassi (D)
Fresh lime for beans (O)
Mint chutney (O)
Tea (have tea 1 hour after lassi) (O)

Chapati/plain rice or saffron rice with
  vegetables (G)
Squash, moon dal kitchari (pitta) or fried
  kidney beans (M)
Carrot halva or pachak lassi or tea (D)
Squeeze of lime (O)
Coriander chutney (O)
Tea (have tea 1 hour after lassi) (O)

Snacks
Coconut cookies (G)
Seasonal fresh fruit (N)
Cool milk with rosewater (D)
Mint tea (O)

Oatmeal cookies (G)
Sweet apple or pear (V)
Hot almond milk or spiced milk with ghee and
  turmeric – best 30 minutes before bed (D)

Dinner
Chapati (G)
Fried rice (G)
Mixed vegetable soup (V)
Roasted, ground sunflower seeds
  to sprinkle on the soup (M)
Fresh lime for the soup (O)
Tea (O)

Chapati or puri (G)
Potato vegetable curry
Lentil soup or egg-white omelette (M)
Squeeze of lime (O)
Agni tea (O)

Ideal menu for kapha

Breakfast
Puffed millet or oat granola (G)
½ cup skimmed goat's milk or soya milk (D)
Kapha tea with 1 teaspoon honey, if desired (O)

Creamed rye or spiced oatmeal porridge (G)
  or suitable fruit (V)
Kapha tea with 1 teaspoon honey, if desired (O)

Lunch
Rye bread (without yeast) or spiced cooked
  millet or barley (G)
Green beans – protein derived from bean and
  grain combination (V) (M)
Fresh lime or lemon (O)
Carrot chutney (O)

Corn tortilla or cornbread (G)
Cabbage – with kitchari (V)
Moong dal kitchari or tofu and vegetables (M)
Fresh lime (O)
Green mango chutney (O)

Snacks
1 or 2 rice cakes (G)
Seasonal fruit or juice (V)
Roasted, unsalted sunflower seeds (M)
1 cup herbal tea with ginger, cinnamon or mint (O)

Popcorn (no salt or butter) or unsalted corn
  chips with salsa (G)
Apples or pears or other seasonal fruit (V)
1 cup herbal tea (O)

Dinner
Mixed green salad with lemon or lime juice (V)
Tapioca kitchari (M)
(Note: grains should not be eaten with tapioca)
Fresh lime or lemon (O)
Turmeric chutney (O)
Agni tea (O)

Rye bread (without yeast) or rye crackers,
  flaky rice with potatoes (G)
Corn soup – protein from corn and rye (V) (M)
Fresh lime (O)
Fresh coriander chutney (O)
Spicy tea (O)

Incompatible food combinations

Within the field of holistic health and nutrition, there is a great deal of controversy about the issue of food combining. Even among the population at large, there is growing concern about diet and confusion over the large number of conflicting theories on the subject.

Ayurveda offers a logical and scientific approach for determining an appropriate diet based upon your prakruti (see pages 28–34), which are determined by your unique combinations of vata, pitta and kapha doshas. This approach is quite different from the 'traditional' view of a balanced diet – eating daily from the basic food groups of meat, dairy, fruit, grains and vegetables. According to ayurveda, such a scheme is not enough to lead us to the goal of good health.

In the classical ayurvedic literature, five types of nutritional disorder have been identified:

- Quantitative dietary deficiency – undernutrition due to insufficient food and even starvation
- Qualitative dietary deficiency – the wrong food combinations, which result in malnutrition, toxic conditions and lack of essential nutrients
- Qualitative and quantitative overnutrition – includes emotional overeating, which can result in obesity and/or high cholesterol, which in turn can lead to hypertension, heart attacks or paralysis
- Toxins in food – certain foods and food combinations lead to toxaemia and digestive disorders
- Unsuitable foods – foods not suitable for your prakruti may affect your natural resistance and cause disease

These five factors are closely connected to the strength of your agni (digestive fire). There are four types of agni:

- *Vishama agni* (erratic internal fire) – This is where the vata dosha is increased, upsetting the balance of your digestive capacity. It causes irregular appetite, indigestion and gas formation. Emotionally, this can result in anxiety, insecurity, fear and neurological or mental problems.
- *Tikshna agni* (hyperactive internal fire) – Pitta dosha is responsible for this type of digestive capacity disorder. It may cause hypermetabolism, hyperacidity, heartburn and hypoglycaemia, leading to inflammatory diseases.
- *Manda agni* (hypoactive, or low, internal fire) – This is due to an excess of kapha, leading to

List of incompatible food combinations

The *Charaka Samhita*, the oldest ayurvedic text, describes a number of incompatible food combinations. The list below provides more suggestions on foods which, in combination, could be harmful to health. This list is by no means complete, nor is it inflexible.

It is important for you, as an individual, to observe the effects of your daily diet on your health. Work out what food combinations make you feel good and what make you sluggish. You can then make the necessary adjustments in order to enhance your sense of wellbeing.

Milk is incompatible with:
- Bananas
- Fish
- Meat
- Melons
- Curd/yogurt
- Sour fruits
- Cherries
- Bread that contains yeast

Melons are incompatible with:
- Grains
- Starch
- Fried foods
- Cheese

Starches are incompatible with:
- Eggs
- Tea
- Milk
- Bananas
- Dates
- Persimmons

Honey is incompatible with:
- Ghee (in equal proportions)
- Heating or cooking

Radishes are incompatible with:
- Milk
- Bananas
- Raisins

Members of the nightshade family (potato, tomato, chillies, aubergine/eggplant, peppers) are incompatible with:
- Yogurt
- Milk
- Melon
- Cucumber

Yogurt is incompatible with:
- Milk
- Sour fruits
- Melons
- Hot drinks
- Meat
- Fish
- Mangoes
- Starch
- Cheese

Eggs are incompatible with:
- Milk
- Meat
- Yogurt
- Melons
- Cheese
- Fish
- Bananas

Mango is incompatible with:
- Yogurt
- Cheese
- Cucumbers

Corn is incompatible with:
- Dates
- Raisins
- Bananas

Lemon is incompatible with:
- Yogurt
- Milk
- Cucumbers
- Tomatoes

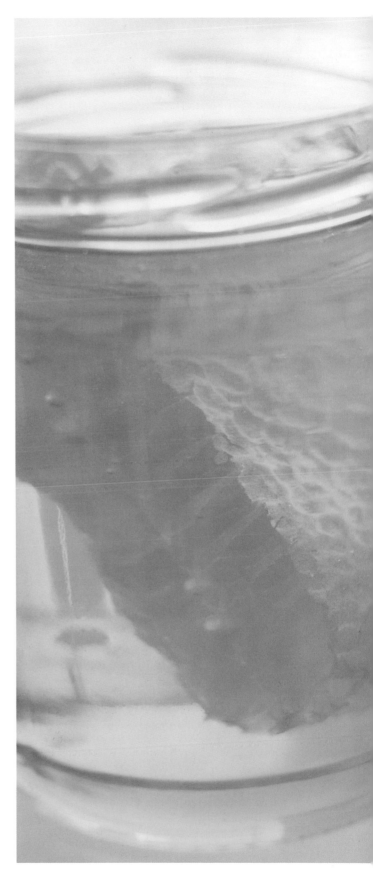

right WHILE RAW HONEY IS AN ACCEPTABLE NATURAL SWEETENER, COOKED HONEY DIGESTS SLOWLY, CLOGS THE BODY'S CHANNELS AND PRODUCES TOXINS

slow metabolism, increased weight or obesity, allergies and congestive diseases.

- *Sama agni* (balanced internal fire) – This type of agni is the result of the three doshas each being in equilibrium. A person with this type of digestive capacity can eat almost any type of food without difficulty. Digestion, absorption and elimination are all normal.

Ayurvedic nutritionists consider these types of agni when making suggestions concerning diet.

According to ayurveda, every food has its own taste, heating or cooling energy and post-digestive effect. When two or three different food substances of different taste, energy and post-digestive effect are combined, the digestive capacity can become overloaded, inhibiting the enzyme system and resulting in the production of toxins in the system. Equally, certain food combinations can slow your digestive capacity. Undigested food then remains in the stomach for seven to eight hours. These same foods, if eaten separately, may well stimulate digestive capacity, be digested more quickly and even help to burn ama.

Combining foods improperly can produce indigestion, fermentation, putrefaction and the formation of gas. This condition, if prolonged, can lead to toxaemia and disease. For example, eating bananas with milk can diminish your digestive capacity, alter the intestinal flora so and produce toxins; this may cause a cold, cough, sinus congestion and allergies.

BASIC FOOD-COMBINING CONCEPTS
- Avoid having milk or yogurt with sour or citrus fruits, such as lemons.
- Avoid eating fruits with potatoes or other starchy foods, such as bread or pasta.
- Avoid eating melons and grains together.
- Honey should never be cooked. Honey digests slowly when cooked and the molecules become like a glue, adhering to mucus membranes and clogging the body's channels, producing toxins. Uncooked honey is nectar. Cooked honey is poison.
- Do not eat meat protein and milk protein together. Meat is heating and milk is cooling, so they counteract one another, disturb digestive capacity and produce ama (improperly digested food).
- Milk and melons should not be eaten together. Both are cooling, but milk is a laxative and melon is diuretic. Milk also requires more time to digest.

Ayurvedic therapies

Disease is an inevitable aspect of life. Any measures designed to ease the disease process are known as therapy (*chikitsa* or *upakrama*). At the core of ayurveda is the necessity to understand the body both in sickness and in health. Its curative methods go beyond employing only medicines or conducting surgery, and it aims to heal the body naturally.

Ayurveda classifies its therapeutic approaches in two ways. Each addresses two specific ayurvedic objectives: preventive healthcare and the process of healing.

Therapies are classified into two main categories:

• Anabolic – *santarpana*
• Catabolic – *apatarpana*

The Sanskrit term *tarpana* refers to the condition of nourishment. Hence *santarpana*, or anabolic therapy, means treatments that nourish our body and its tissues. This invariably results in promoting bulk and weight. Enhancing earth and water elements in your body, through drugs or diet, makes this possible. In contrast, *apatarpana*, or catabolic therapy, is a process by which your body is deprived of or given less nourishment – although, crucially, not the essential nutrients. This helps you to lose weight and bulk, and is achieved by using elements such as space, air and fire. The catabolic therapies fall into the following categories: purifying or eliminative (*shodhana*) and restorative or palliative (*shamana*).

In the *Charak Samhita*, six therapies are mentioned:

• *Langhana* – treatment which causes lightness or reduces the size of the body
• *Bramhana* – treatment which increases the size of the body and makes it stronger
• *Rukshana* – treatment which produces dryness, roughness and clearness
• *Snehana* – treatment which increases viscosity, fluidity, softness and moistness in the body, oil therapy (see pages 54 and 57)
• *Swedana* – treatment which causes perspiration and destroys stiffness, heaviness and coldness in the body, sweating therapy (see pages 54 and 57)
• *Sthambhana* – treatment which blocks, stops, holds, retards and stabilizes whatever flows within the body

These therapies may be used in combination depending upon the disease or diseases from which you are suffering. If administered judiciously and correctly by a qualified ayurvedic physician, with due regard to dosage and season, they can cure or alleviate all the 'curable' ailments from which we, as humans, suffer.

Preventive therapies

While it is true that all the therapies described above are used when you are suffering from disease – and are therefore known as curative therapies – ayurveda also has an important preventive role. While the main aim in treating any ailment is to relieve pain and suffering, it is also important to establish good health. The process should not only cure you of illness or disease, but also increase your resistance or immunity to that ailment in the future. This is the aim of the preventive therapies: rejuvenation therapy (see page 86) and virilification therapy (page 87). It is best to undertake these after an illness or when you are apparently healthy.

Life span or longevity

Our individual life span depends upon two factors: the unseen (God or the Divine) and the seen (controllable, human factors). The unseen (*daiva*) is predetermined, and it is the result of the deeds of your previous life. The seen (*purushakara*) is within your control and is your conduct in your present life. All of us would like to live long and happy lives. There are three seen factors involved in increasing longevity:

• A balanced inheritance – that is, the quality of sperm and ovum, prenatal and neonatal care and the physical and mental wellbeing of both parents at the time of conception
• Having a good quality of spirit – following a righteous life and avoiding envy, materialism, greed and selfishness
• Adopting a good diet and healthy lifestyle

Ageing

Two of the best-known theories of ageing are:

• The programmed ageing theory
• The wear and tear theory

THE PROGRAMMED AGEING THEORY
According to ayurveda, the body degenerates and decays itself. Like a clock that slowly unwinds, so the body ages in accordance with a normal development pattern built into every organism. This programme is preset for each individual and is beyond human control. It is your karma. This is primary ageing and accords with the unseen factor (*daiva*) that controls our life span.

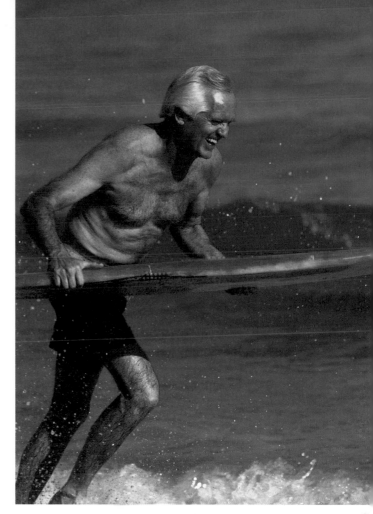

The three doshas are responsible for health and disease, and are predominant in each phase of life irrespective of your prakruti. According to this theory, the first phase of life is dominated by kapha, the second by pitta and the third and last phase by vata. Similarly, over the period of your life, there is gross degeneration of the vital energy (*ojas*), that is responsible for resistance, immunity and wellbeing. The ojas within our bodies is formed by the seven body tissues (*dhatus*). As a general rule, every change that takes place in your body and mind as part of the ageing process can be attributed to aggravated vata and deteriorated ojas.

- There is a gradual decline in the fives senses as we age. The lens of the eyes, for instance, become less elastic with age, so that focus is slow to adjust. As a result, many people develop presbyopia – farsightedness associated with ageing – and need glasses. Sensitivity of smell, on the other hand, holds up well; it is one of the last senses to decline.
- Older people have fewer tastebuds and their olfactory bulb is withered, so that food seems to have less taste. They tend to eat less and are often undernourished.
- The ability to handle new material or situations typically declines with age, while the ability to solve problems on the basis of automatic processing of stored information does not.
- Older people are less efficient at encoding information – that is, preparing and labelling it for storage so that is easier to retrieve when needed.
- The stability of body declines. Muscles sag and emaciate. Veins become prominent.
- There is a shift from an outward orientation, or a concern with finding a place in society, to an inward one, a search for meaning within the self. This may be unsettling. Many people feel a need to participate in and guide the next generation. If this is not met, they stagnate and become lifeless.
- Many older people suffer from a variety of more or less disabling aches and pains; some have lost spouses, siblings, friends and even children. They may take medications that cause mood alterations and feel that they have no control over their lives. At any given time, about one-third of those who are over 65 suffer from depression. Depressed people tend to be become disorganized, absent-minded, careless, apathetic, unable to concentrate and uninterested in the world around them.
- Wrinkles, baldness, lack of proper sleep, affinity to heat and constipation are some of the direct effects of vata predominance and ojas depletion as we age.
- The most common conditions in older people are arthritis, hypertension, heart disease, cataracts, impairments of legs, hips, back or spine – all of which are attributable to aggravated vata.

THE WEAR AND TEAR THEORY

This relates to secondary ageing and correlates to the seen, or controllable, factor of our life span. The body ages because of continuous use, abuse, disuse and disease. Muscles become flabby, joints deteriorate, and accumulated excess fat liquifies. When people age, the marrow does not remain intact inside the bones, there is impairment in the ejaculation of semen in males and the ojas, or vital energy, declines. Older people feel exhausted and languid, and succumb to excess sleep, drowsiness and laziness. They lose initiative, have difficulty catching their breath and become incapable of physical and mental work. They also suffer from memory loss, impaired intellect and a deteriorating complexion, and become susceptible to disease. This is why older people should give up any unwholesome dietary or other lifestyle habits, and undergo rejuvenation therapy (*rasayana*). Rasayana is ayurveda's answer to controlling the ageing process and promoting an active, long-lasting life (see page 86).

Yoga

Originating in India several thousand years ago, the practice of yoga today has devotees all over the world. It is an intrinsic part of ayurveda, and the use of yoga and yoga therapy for treating illness and improving health and general wellbeing is a common part of all ayurvedic treatment and philosophy. In fact, ayurveda originates from the six schools of Hindu philosophy known as the *Shaddharsanas*. These are:

• Samkhya
• Yoga
• Nyaya
• Vaiseshika
• Vedanta
• Mimasma

Of these six, the first four are strongly connected to ayurveda.

In the West, there is the rather curious practice of labelling yoga by various 'brand' names such as ashtanga or iyengar. True practitioners of this ancient knowledge see this branding as superfluous and simply an attempt to attach importance to the particular school of yoga which you have chosen. Rather, its importance is as a method of achieving spiritual harmony through control of your mind and body.

The eight steps involved in yoga are:

• Yama – control of the senses
• Niyama – restrictions on behaviour
• Asana – correct posture
• Pranayama – breathing
• Pratyaha – withdrawal from the sensory world
• Dharana – awareness of the self
• Dhyana – meditation
• Samadhi – oneness with God/ super-consciousness

The true purpose of yoga is to 'yoke' or unite the individual soul to the cosmic soul. In the process of that journey, you can also use yoga to achieve good health. Additionally, the asanas (yogic postures) and pranayama (breath control) help us to develop the inner strength to deal with life's stresses and strains serenely and calmly.

Sometimes, people who take up yoga initially find it difficult because of their physical or mental conditioning. However, practising yoga in conjunction with ayurvedic treatment is an extremely powerful tool in curing disease, particularly in cases of:

• Rheumatism and rheumatoid arthritis
• Back pain
• Migraine
• Depression
• Sinus problems

The Ayurvedic Charitable Hospital in London (see page 126) has worked in conjunction with the excellent therapists from the Yoga Biomedical Trust to offer this form of treatment to its patients. These patients have benefited significantly from the highly effective combination of yoga and ayurveda.

The Sanskrit word *asana* means 'to seat oneself in a comfortable position'. Yogic positions (asanas) that are ideal for some common health problems are:

• Padimasana – the lotus position
• Siddhasana – posture of the adept
• Paschimottanasana – stretching the back and hips
  • Bhujangasana – the cobra position
    • Savasana – the complete relaxation posture

The asanas help to relax both the body and the mind. They not only improve muscle tone, but also have a healing effect on the body's internal organs. Your circulation and digestion will improve, and there are also positive benefits for your respiratory, reproductive, nervous and endocrine systems.

Ideally, the asanas should be followed by the practice of yogic breathing, or pranayama. It is also important to remember that postures should be chosen which take your prakruti, or physical constitution, into consideration. A properly qualified yoga teacher or your ayurvedic practitioner should be able to help you with this.

Yoga is a wonderful system of exercise. This gentle method of achieving physical, mental and emotional balance can be practised by anyone, regardless of

left and right **YOGA IS A WONDERFUL EXERCISE FOR THE BODY AND THE MIND, LEAVING YOU SUPPLE AND FLEXIBLE, STRONG AND CALM. THE POSTURES (ASANAS) SHOWN HERE ARE: RAISED TADASANA (LEFT), ARDHO MUKHA SVANASANA, OR DOWNWARD DOG (ABOVE RIGHT), AND URDHVA MUKHA SVANASANA, OR UPWARD DOG (RIGHT)**

their age, sex, level of fitness and flexibility. Once you have mastered the basic postures, you can build them into your daily routine, and they can be done anywhere. Never strain or force your body when performing asanas, and always rest if you start to feel tired. Do each asana slowly, patiently and carefully – otherwise the effects will be negative. Remain conscious of your breathing throughout and never hold your breath. Yoga is done to best advantage early in the morning or late afternoon.

Pranayama

Pranayama, or yogic breathing, burns up karma, and those who practice it will find that their spiritual potential will be awakened very quickly. They will become more spiritual, with a sharper memory and a higher sensitivity. In fact, if you take up pranayama, you may notice that, in the first few months after starting to practice this form of breathing, you feel more acutely free from the pain of your fellow human beings and your own suffering. However, this feeling will soon pass and you will come to possess improved awareness of and detachment from your selfish concerns and a greater sense of equanimity.

Although breathing is an autonomic reflex, most of us in fact do not breathe correctly. We usually perform the act without conscious thought and without proper appreciation of its effects within our bodies. Yet our health depends upon our ability to breathe properly. Utilizing our lung capacity to its fullest extent helps to combat fatigue, headaches and lack of concentration, among other things.

Pranayama is a Sanskrit term made up of the two words *prana* (life force, or the breath of life) and *yama* (control). Hence it is all about breathing with control and in the correct fashion. The techniques of yogic breathing involve using the downward movement of the diaphragm (the layer of muscle that separates the lung from the stomach) as you breathe in such a way as to expand the lungs downwards, taking in more air than they normally do. This helps to oxygenate the lower part of the lungs and cleanse it of mucus and impurities. It is this process that particularly helps people who suffer from asthma, bronchitis and chronic lung problems.

Pranayama is a serious and highly spiritual practice. It should only be carried out under the expert guidance and supervision of a trained, advanced yoga instructor or spiritual guru. Always consult a qualified, competent yoga teacher if you wish to take up pranayama, or even yoga in general, as it is extremely ill advised to try to learn these practices from simply reading a book.

BENEFITS OF PRANAYAMA

Pranayama, or the science of breathing, helps us to tap into the vital energy stored within our bodies. The proper practice of pranayama can show significant benefits for the following conditions:

- Asthma or bronchitis
- Sinus problems
- Ear, nose or throat infections
- Eczema
- High blood pressure
- Obesity

Meditation

Meditation is truly the 'cleansing of consciousness' and the heightening of awareness – the ultimate state achieved through yoga. In fact, the entire purpose of the eightfold yogic path is to achieve the states of awareness (*dharana*), meditation (*dhyana*) and oneness with God or the superconscious (samadhi). It is not simply about reducing weight or looking good.

During the process of meditation, your mind is cleansed of all thought processes and the residual attachments, insecurities and fears that dog all human existence. In Hindu philosophical terms, the mind is simply the crust of the soul that carries information from the five senses. As Lord Krishna says in the *Gita,* his seven-hundred verse instruction towards self-realization, 'The mind enslaved by the five senses the mind is the servant of the material world.' The soul, on the other hand, is eternal, and its essential nature is knowledge and bliss. The mind, which is the repository of the ego, is the product of karma and the environment.

The process of meditation

How do you meditate? What is the correct way to meditate? What will meditation do for me? These are the types of question all seekers of peace ask.

Ideally, all meditation should be taught by a guru or a teacher who has been initiated or is part of the ancient and venerable tradition of *Tapas* (renunciation, or meditation). Meditation can be done:

- On the breath
- On visual images
- On mantras
- On yantras (mandalas or geometric patterns)

Position is important in meditation. As one aim of meditation is to achieve slower and more even breathing, it is important to sit in a comfortable position with your spine straight, preferably in the lotus position of yoga or with your legs crossed in a comfortable position (*sukhasana*). Do not slouch or sit in a cramped fashion. Air should be able to flow in and out of your lungs freely and without impediment.

You can simply 'watch' the breath as it flows through your nostrils and into your lungs and then notice it turn as you breathe out. There is a famous 'mantra' of this inflowing and outflowing breath that is the essence of the Hindu tradition. Unfortunately, it is against the principles of the author to write 'mantras' in books, but those who want to learn it should feel free to contact him at the telephone number given in the Directory (page 126), and it will be taught free of charge at the appropriate time for the seeker.

Meditating on a mantra is an age-old practice in India and, correctly initiated by a guru, the mantra is the 'vehicle' that will transport the seeker through the ocean of life with greater ease. Mantras are an integral facet of ayurveda, and can be used to treat serious and chronic illnesses. Yantras, or geometric patterns, are also used for meditation, including the Sri yantra. The combination of mantra and yantra in meditation is the most powerful of all practices, one which in fact awakens miraculous powers, or *Siddhis*. Seeking these miraculous powers deliberately, as the reward of meditation, is considered quite wrong and is only done by those with ignoble intentions.

In some Buddhist practices, particularly Vajrayana Buddhism, it is a tradition to meditate on the third eye in the forehead, visualizing a white dot or an aura.

The goal of all meditation should be the calming and purification of your mind and your actions. It is not necessary, or even desirable, to empty your mind of all thoughts. Rather, the aim is to let your thoughts flow naturally until you reach a place of peace. Allow thoughts to enter your mind, then simply let them go.

The benefits of meditation

Scientific studies are not the criteria by which the benefits of meditation are judged by the evolved soul. However, for the sake of the sceptics, there are scientifically evaluated benefits, including:

- The lowering of high blood pressure (hypertension)
- Release from tension and stress
- Freedom from anxiety
- Reduction of migraine and headache
- Improved immunity
- Better and more restful sleep
- Improved self-esteem and confidence
- Heightened intelligence and creativity

In ayurvedic terms, meditation has a valuable role to play in keeping your doshas in balance. Above all, though, meditation is about improving your mental, physical and spiritual wellbeing.

right **MEDITATION CAN BE PRACTISED ANYWHERE TO CALM AND PURIFY THE MIND. SIT UP STRAIGHT AND COMFORTABLY SO THAT YOUR BREATHING IS DEEP AND STEADY, AND LET YOUR THOUGHTS FLOW NATURALLY UNTIL YOU REACH A STATE OF PEACE**

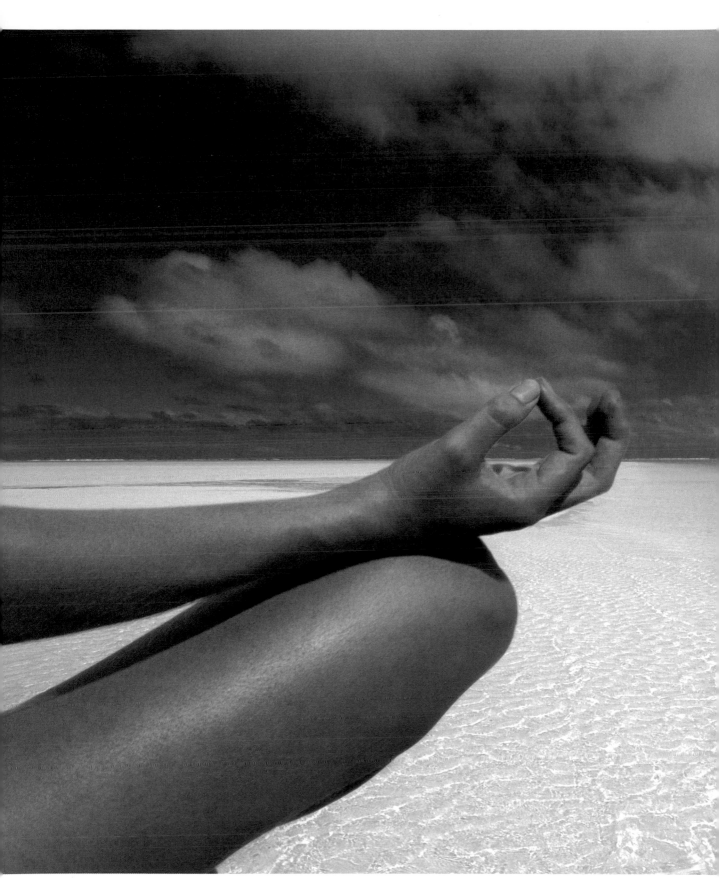

Rejuvenation therapy

According to Charaka, anyone of normal faculty, intelligence, strength and energy, who is desirous of his wellbeing pertaining to this world and the world beyond, has to seek three basic desires: the desire to live, the desire to earn a living and the desire to perform virtuous acts. The desire to live is the chief among the three, as everything ends with the end of life. Everybody wants to live longer, but nobody wants to grow old. However, we cannot attain immortality because we are bound by the rules of our organic constitutions, but we can improve the quality of our lives with rejuvenation therapy.

Rejuvenation therapy, or *rasayana*, affects the body and the mind simultaneously and brings about a physical and psychological improvement. It prevents the effects of early ageing on both the mind and the body, and increases the body's resistance to disease.

In ayurveda, any drug, diet or conduct that enlivens your body and mind is considered rejuvenation therapy. Rejuvenation therapy also prevents disease. There are a number of ayurvedic drugs and substances that possess the qualities of maintaining health, prolonging life and warding off disease. They are all grouped as rejuvenation therapy in ayurveda.

- The qualitative, quantitative and functional balance of the body elements maintains strength, which in general causes resistance to disease. Great importance is attached to your blood, as its normal condition reflects good health and general resistance to disease.
- In ayurveda, a separate substance known as ojas (vital energy) is described and is said to be the essence of all the body tissues. A vital body element, ojas is the condition or excellence of the body as a whole. Resistance depends on the quality and quantity of ojas.
- Strength or power (*bala*) has been classified as natural or hereditary (*sahaja*), variable according to age and season (*kalakrita*) and acquired by good diet, medicines and exercise (*yuktikrita*). This is why some families have a resistance to specific diseases; some diseases manifest at a particular age or season, and, generally speaking, those who are well built are less likely to fall ill.
- Researchers have proven that rejuvenation therapy increases blood levels of gamma globulins, indicating an increase in non-specific resistance. Disease sets in only when your body becomes weak and the offending agent or

substance becomes strong and weakens your body's overall condition, or ojas. All rejuvenation treatments are therefore targeted at improving your ojas, immunity and resistance.

Before undergoing rejuvenation therapy, you need to go through the process of panchakarma, or purification therapy (see pages 56–62).

Behavioural rejuvenation therapy

There are many activities that promote happiness and a healthy body. These are known as behavioural rasayanas (*achara rasayana*). They strengthen life by stimulating and creating positive emotions and experiences, which in turn promote the production of ojas, a vital substance that creates balance and health in our physiology. Refined emotions and a positive, loving approach to life are qualities that develop over time, from the inside out, through deep integration of mind and body. The most important trigger of this process is the regular experience of pure consciousness.

Ayurvedic texts give a number of such behavioural rasayanas. Some of them are listed below:

INTERPERSONAL RELATIONS
- Do not entertain negativity such as anger, hostility, cynicism and indignation.
- If a negative feeling comes up, let it go. It is in the letting go that our choice lies.
- Invest your energy in thoughts and actions that help the growth of positivity and, whenever possible, make a choice for happiness. Bliss is the best recipe for eliminating mental ama (toxins).
- Keep the company of the wise.
- Choose to be with those who uplift and inspire you and lead you to strive for greater knowledge, consideration of others, charity and wisdom.

SPEECH
- Speak the truth, but speak it sweetly.
- Speaking the truth discourages deviousness, deceit and other mental modes that complicate and muddle the mind.
- Maintain personal integrity, which enhances self-esteem and self-confidence.

CLEANLINESS
Maintain cleanliness in all things – mental, physical and environmental. Maintaining a clean, dignified and beautiful environment will uplift and inspire the mind, resulting in the creation of positive emotions and sense of comfort and wellbeing that are health-inducing.

CHARITY
- Be charitable in all areas of life.
- Adopt an attitude of giving.
- Donate money, knowledge, advice and encouragement.

SPIRITUALITY
Follow the precepts of your own spiritual beliefs, devoting time for spiritual practices that appeal to you. This provides a beautiful channel for the heart to flow and your devotional nature to unfold. We all learn to surrender to the supreme being or intelligence as we practice spirituality, and this is probably the most blissful experience we may have in our life.

Virilification therapy

Virilification therapy (*vajikarana*), like rejuvenation therapy, is an important branch of ayurveda. The main aim of virilification therapy is to improve both the function and the health of the reproductive tissues. Healthy parents have healthy offspring. Ayurveda has always emphasized that, for perfectly healthy progeny,

the parents' health must be good – particularly their sexual health. This is enhanced through virilification therapy. There are several herbal medicines described in ayurveda that have potent effects on virility. Some of these herbs also qualify as rejuvenating.

Hindu culture has always upheld the principles of abstinence. Virilification therapy's original intention was never to exploit sex for pleasure; it is simply meant to engender a sound and tenacious sperm and ovum in order to produce a healthy child. Although, according to ayurvedic principles, sexual drives must be regulated and sublimated to realizing the higher purposes in life, views on celibacy and abstinence have relaxed somewhat. Today, virilification therapy is used to treat conditions such as stress-related impotence. Still, ayurveda cautions physicians against misuse of both rejuvenation and virilification therapies. Also, before any treatment can be carried out, panchakarma must be undertaken (see pages 56–62).

below **VIRILIFICATION THERAPY AIMS TO IMPROVE YOUR SEXUAL OR REPRODUCTIVE HEALTH SO THAT ANY CHILD YOU HAVE IS GIVEN THE BEST POSSIBLE START IN LIFE**

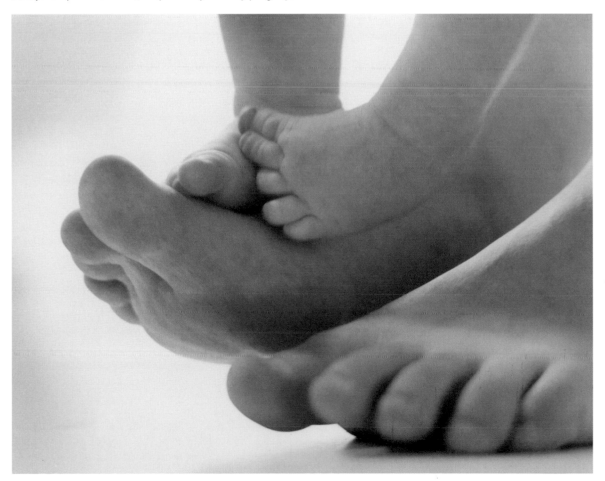

Ayurveda and astrology

Ayurveda and astrology are strongly linked and part of the traditional Hindu approach to life. Astrologers are consulted about ill health, marriages, career matters and all aspects of the lives of the ordinary Indian.

Ayurvedic teachings emphasize that all diseases are the product of karma, or 'destiny'. Astrology is the barometer of an individual's karma and the birth chart will clearly indicate the progress of a disease and whether or not it is curable. Few ayurvedic physicians may nowadays make or refer to your astrological chart, but those who do so with good knowledge of both ayurveda and astrology can be of great help, particularly if you are suffering from a major illness.

The 12 signs of the zodiac, the nine planets and their movements through the signs, and the lunar constellations in the zodiac signs together form the basis of Vedic astrology (jyotish). The influence of the moon is considered very important. It even has a bearing on your individual constitution, or prakruti. The 12 signs and 27 lunar constellations are shown opposite in a typical jyotish chart, while the table below shows the 27 stars, the houses they occupy and the prakruti, or doshic constitution, they influence.

Treatments are best started and carried out on certain days and avoided on other days. As ayurveda does not cater for emergency cases as a rule, it is relatively easy to ensure that this happens. Obviously, emergency cases such as accident or heart attack victims cannot adhere to this.

If you are undergoing the 7½-year period of Saturn (known as Sade Sathi), when the planet Saturn moves through the twelfth, first and second house to the position of the moon at birth (called the natal moon), you may find that illnesses linger despite all treatment. Planets in a bad position can cause major illnesses, particularly if they are the maleficent planets such as Saturn or Mars, the Sun or the nodes Rahu and Ketu.

On days when the moon is transiting the eighth house to the position of moon at birth, starting treatment or undergoing major procedures should be avoided. In other words, if the moon was in Aries when you were born, serious treatment should be avoided when the moon is in Scorpio. This is known as Chandvashtama (eighth house moon).

The 27 stars also relate to the three gunas that classify humans into satvic (spiritual), rajasic (human) and tamasic (materialistic) types (see page 35).

Under the guidance of a wise astrologer who is also an ayurvedic physician, you can gain great insight into the karmic causes of your illness, and progress dramatically both physically and spiritually.

The 27 stars of Hindu astrology

VATA STAR	ZODIAC SIGN LOCATED IN	PITTA STAR	ZODIAC SIGN LOCATED IN	KAPHA STAR	ZODIAC SIGN LOCATED IN
Krittika	Aries/Taurus	Bharani	Aries	Aswini	Aries
Ashlesha	Cancer	Rohini	Taurus	Mrigashira	Taurus/Gemini
Makha	Leo	Ardra	Gemini	Punarvasu	Gemini
Chaitra	Virgo/Leo	Pubba	Leo	Pushya	Cancer
Visakha	Libra/Scorpio	Uttura Phalguni	Leo/Virgo	Hasta	Virgo
Jyeshta	Scorpio	Poorvashadha	Sagittarius	Swati	Libra
Moola	Sagittarius	Uttarashadha	Sagittarius/ Capricorn	Anuradha	Scorpio
Dhanishta	Capricorn	Poorva Bhadrapada	Aquarius/Pisces	Sravana	Capricorn
Satabhisha	Aquarius	Uttra Bhadrapada	Pisces	Revati	Pisces

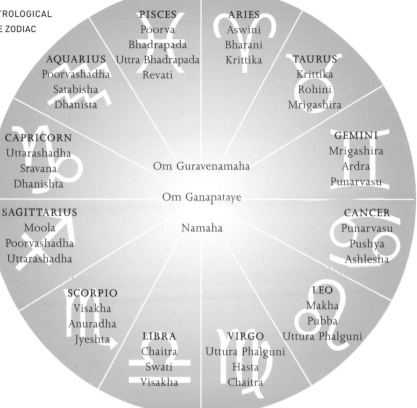

PISCES
Poorva
Bhadrapada
Uttra Bhadrapada
Revati

ARIES
Aswini
Bharani
Krittika

AQUARIUS
Poorvashadha
Satabisha
Dhanista

TAURUS
Krittika
Rohini
Mrigashira

CAPRICORN
Uttarashadha
Sravana
Dhanishta

GEMINI
Mrigashira
Ardra
Punarvasu

Om Guravenamaha

Om Ganapataye

Namaha

SAGITTARIUS
Moola
Poorvashadha
Uttarashadha

CANCER
Punarvasu
Pushya
Ashlesha

SCORPIO
Visakha
Anuradha
Jyeshta

LEO
Makha
Pubba
Uttura Phalguni

LIBRA
Chaitra
Swati
Visakha

VIRGO
Uttura Phalguni
Hasta
Chaitra

Diseases caused by planets in difficult positions

MARS
Unfavourable Mars can cause a variety of illnesses, including digestive problems. Wearing corals may help.

VENUS
Venus can cause gynaecological and sexual diseases. Diamond is the gemstone for countering Venus.

MERCURY
Mercury causes many ailments, including high blood pressure. Emerald is the gem for Mercury.

JUPITER
Jupiter causes obesity and urinary problems. Topaz is the gemstone for this planet.

SATURN
Saturn can cause a variety of ailments and sorrow. Dark blue sapphire is the stone for Saturn.

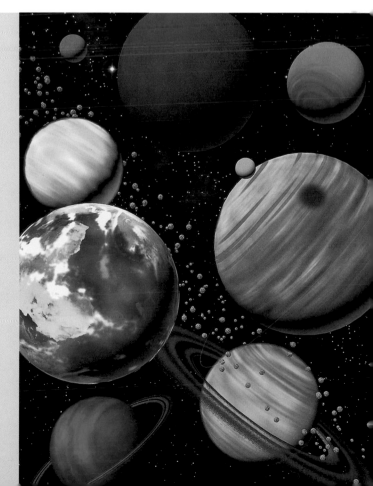

right IN AYURVEDA, THE PLANETS AND THEIR MOVEMENTS HAVE A PROFOUND EFFECT ON DISEASE AND WELLBEING

Chakra and marma therapy

There is no topic on which the author of this book feel as strongly as the increasing misuse of so-called chakra and marma therapy.

Chakra and marma therapy are not part of traditional ayurvedic treatment. They are, in fact, extremely delicate and potentially dangerous practices which can have very serious consequences, including madness or death, for someone who is a victim of a charlatan claiming expertise in these esoteric techniques.

Marma therapy is often practised by acupuncturists who falsely claim proper knowledge of ayurveda, but do not have any idea of the ayurvedic detoxification technique of panchakarma (see pages 56–62) or of the vast number of plants and medications that are part of the panchakarma procedures.

Marmas, according to ayurveda, are extremely sensitive nerve points which should be guarded from injury at any cost and are not to be punctured as in acupuncture. They are different from the points used in acupuncture for treatment with needles. These nerve points, according to the ayurvedic texts, can at best be gently massaged using light pressure by highly experienced marma experts, These experts are more often than not martial arts experts trained to avoid injury to these vital parts.

Chakra therapy is even more dangerous and must be avoided completely. Chakras should be left well alone and, if they are to be opened, they will do so naturally as a result of years of *sadhana* (deep meditation) under the guidance of a realized guru. All attempts to awaken the kundalini or the chakras either by the self or by the growing army of New Age chakra healers are bound to end in serious trouble for the seeker. The basic precept in all kundalini-related knowledge is that it takes lifetimes to open a chakra and that any forced attempt, either by a healer or by a therapist, to do so will result in serious mental and physical disturbances.

You are strongly advised to avoid all those who seek to offer marma therapy or give training that will open your chakras or the kundalini, as it can only end in disaster. Just as wise and responsible neuro-surgeons hesitate to operate on the spinal cord due to the dangers of total paralysis, so the teacher who knows that the spinal column is the path of the kundalini will avoid interfering with this vital canal.

Gem therapy

The art of using gems and stones for ayurvedic treatment and astrological purposes has existed in India for more than 7,000 years. Vedic astrology has clear guidelines on the use of gems for curing the diseases and sorrows that plague humans due to the ill effects of planets in malevolent positions. The wearing of gems can help us to reduce the impact of planet-related afflictions on our bodies (see page 89). The nine planets are represented by the *navaratha* (nine gems) as shown in the table opposite, top left.

Gemstones are also linked to ayurveda through their correlation to the five elements of earth, water, fire, air and space. If you are of a predominantly pitta (fire) constitution, for example, you should obviously not wear a ruby as it would increase the heat in an already heated system. Similarly, pearls are not advisable for someone who is a strong kapha type, as they increase water retention and obesity.

Gems can be used to cure illnesses or the ill effects of planetary movements, as shown in the bottom table opposite. Gemstones for an individual are selected on the basis of your date of birth, lunar positions, ascendant, planetary positions and periods. This can only be done by a skilled ayurvedic astrologer. In general, however, the gems listed in the table opposite top right are beneficial for the individual zodiac signs (chosen simply by birth date alone) and should bring good results if an astrologer cannot be consulted

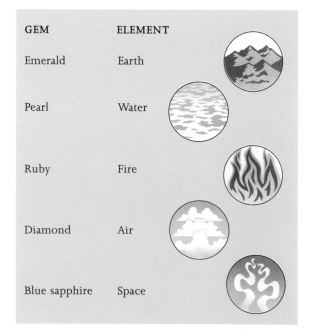

GEM	ELEMENT
Emerald	Earth
Pearl	Water
Ruby	Fire
Diamond	Air
Blue sapphire	Space

Planets & the nine gems

PLANET	GEMSTONE
Mars	Red coral
Sun	Ruby
Jupiter	Yellow sapphire, topaz
Mercury	Emerald
Venus	Diamond
Moon	Pearl
Saturn	Blue sapphire
Rahu	Hessonite
Ketu	Cat's eye

The zodiac & gemstones

ZODIAC SIGN	GEMSTONE	SYMBOLISM
Aries	Blood stone	Courage
Taurus	Diamond	Innocence
Gemini	Emerald	Love
Cancer	Pearl	Health
Leo	Ruby	Contentment
Virgo	Sardonyx	Marital happiness
Libra	Blue sapphire	Spirituality
Scorpio	Opal	Hope
Sagittarius	Yellow sapphire	Fidelity
Capricorn	Turquoise	Prosperity
Aquarius	Garnet	Consistency
Pisces	Amethyst	Sincerity

Disease, healing gemstones & their planetary rulers

DISEASE	APPROPRIATE GEMSTONES	PLANET
Rheumatism, musculoskeletal problems, bone diseases	Red coral, emerald, pearl, dark blue sapphire, ruby	Mars, Mercury, Moon, Saturn, Sun
Digestive diseases, including diabetes	Red coral, white coral, emerald	Mars, Mercury
Diseases of the nervous system	Dark blue sapphire	Saturn, Ketu
Psychological diseases, including hysteria	Emerald in the night, red coral in the day	Mercury, Mars, Ketu
Skin diseases	White coral, yellow sapphire	Mars, Saturn, Rahu
Urinary and gynaecological problems	Pearl, diamond, red coral, yellow sapphire, emerald, topaz	Moon, Venus, Mars, Saturn, Mercury, Jupiter
Dental problems	Sapphire, red coral	Saturn, Mars
Ear, nose and throat problems	Yellow sapphire, white coral	Saturn, Mars
Blood-related problems	Dark blue sapphire, emerald, ruby	Saturn, Mercury, Sun, Rahu

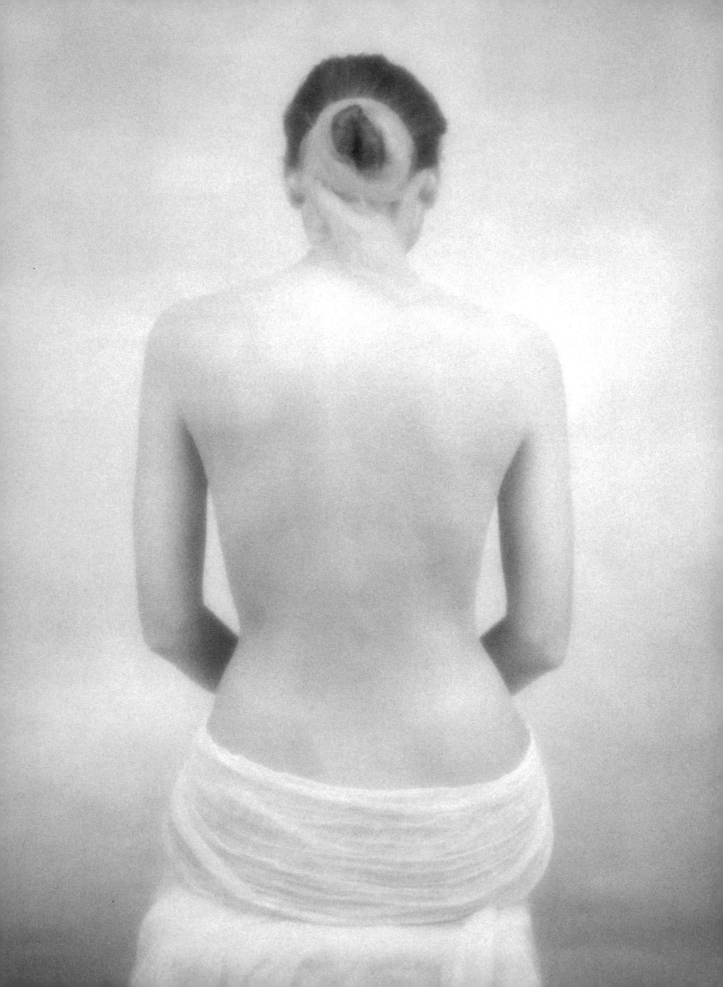

5 cures for common ailments

In ayurveda, every individual is treated as a unique combination of traits, and no ayurvedic treatment is ever the same for all patients, even those suffering the same complaints. This is because, even though two patients may have arthritis, for example, their respective dosha combinations may be so different that the treatment regime will necessarily also be different. While one person may receive panchakarma, appropriate to their age, and the seriousness of the complaint, another may simply be prescribed ayurvedic medicine. It is therefore vitally important that you *always* consult an ayurvedic doctor before taking any of the medication prescribed for the ailments given on the following pages.

Diseases of the digestive system

The group of organs concerned with the ingestion of food, digestion, separation of nutrients and waste products, and absorption of nutrients, is known as *annavaha srotas* in ayurveda. From its beginning to its end, that is, from the mouth to the anus, the digestive tract is a continuous tube of irregular shape and size. The organs included in this system can be classified as follows:

In the head and neck
• Mouth – including the lips
• Teeth
• Palate
• Throat

In the chest
• Oesophagus

In the abdomen
• Stomach
• Duodenum
• Small bowels (intestines)
• Large bowels, colon (intestines)
• Rectum
• Anus

Your liver, gall bladder and pancreas are organs outside this tube, but are connected to it by means of thin ducts. The main function of the digestive system is to receive, digest and absorb food. The ayurvedic view is that the body itself is a product of food and that life is sustained when food is properly utilized. For this reason, food, or nutrition, is considered as one of the three pillars of life (*upasthambha*). The other two pillars are sleep and sex, and spirituality.

The living body is constantly disintegrating and its tissues reduced and converted into energy (*prana*). The food that you eat makes up for these losses and helps in the development of your body's tissues (see page 18) and your body as a whole.

The *prana vayu* (the life force, or inward breath of air) first holds food in your mouth and does not allow it to fall out. It then pushes the food down your gullet. The food then collects in your stomach, where it is moistened and further broken up by the action of *kledaka kapha*, one of the subdoshas of kapha. This converts the food into a soft pulp, which then gradually travels to the duodenum. The *samana vayu* (the equalizing air which governs digestion) now stirs up and excites your body's digestive capacity, or internal fire (*agni*), which in due course, properly digests the food. During digestion, food is broken down into two

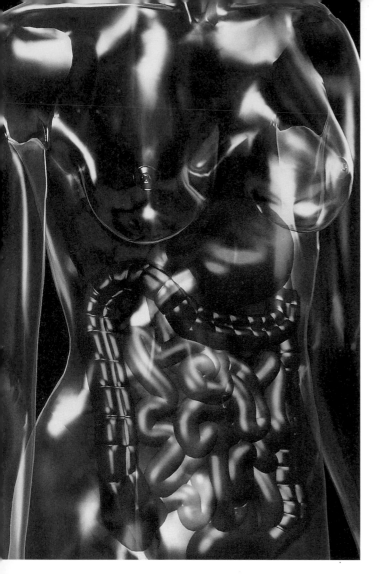

According to ayurveda, the following six factors are responsible for the proper digestion of food:

- Heat
- Movement
- Fluidity, water
- Time
- Oiliness/lubrication
- The excellence and cohesion of all these factors

During digestion, food undergoes three different stages: *madhura avasthà paraka*, which strengthens the kapha dosha; *amla avastha paraka*, which strengthens pitta; and *katu avastha paraka*, which strengthens vata. Thus, the bio-regulating factors of vata, pitta and kapha – the three doshas – are also formed and strengthened during digestion.

GASTRITIS

Many people in today's modern world suffer from gastritis (*amlapitta*) to a lesser or greater degree. In ayurveda, this syndrome is described in some complexity. Gastritis can be the result of a lifestyle change and/or environment and stress.

What causes gastritis?

The main cause of gastritis is unbalanced pitta, which can be aggravated by:

- Eating to excess
- Food which is very hot, astringent, very sour or salty
- Food which causes a burning sensation
- Anger
- Fear
- Excessive exposure to the sun or heat
- Exhaustion
- Eating dry and stale vegetables or incompatible foods, for example milk and fish or milk and radish (see pages 78–9)

What are the symptoms?

Food becomes fermented in the gut as a result of excessive acidity. This fermentation is usually as a result of a high intake of pungent food, as well as an increase of pitta.

parts: useful nutrients and waste products. The nutrients are absorbed and converted into the seven body tissues (*dhatus*), successively from plasma to reproductive tissues (see pages 18), while the waste products are eliminated periodically, keeping your body free of wastes and toxins (*ama*).

All food is made up of the five basic elements of the universe, just as your body is made up of these same five elements. Digestive capacity, or internal fire (*agni*), helps your body to utilize the five basic elements found in food, transforming them into bodily basic elements through the process of digestion. Properly balanced digestive capacity efficiently digests food, thereby effectively nourishing your body. If your digestive capacity is not functioning correctly, it adds to disturbance or imbalance in your three doshas, which in turn leads to disease. It is therefore vital to take care of your digestive capacity, rather than simply focussing specifically on the nutrient value of the food you eat or the amount of calories it contains. Most diseases can in fact be traced back to poor digestive capacity.

In ayurveda, there are two clinical varieties of gastritis:

- Urdhwagata
- Ardhogata

The main symptoms are:

- Indigestion
- Heartburn
- Nausea and lack of appetite
- A feeling of fullness in the stomach
- Pain in the abdomen
- Headache or a heavy feeling in the head
- Sounds in the abdomen
- Loose bowel motions

In the urdhwagata type of gastritis, the following symptoms are also present:

- Vomiting ingested food almost immediately
- A salty, sour, bitter taste in the mouth
- An itching, burning rash on the skin

What is the treatment?

As far as possible, it is important to avoid all factors that can cause or contribute to gastritis

DIETARY FACTORS
Foods to eat: milk, coconut water, dishes containing barley and wheat, bitter vegetables (for example, aubergine/eggplant, Brussels sprouts, spinach), rice with sugar and honey.

Foods to avoid: chillies, hot spices, sour vegetables and fruits, such as tomatoes and citrus fruits, and pungent foods, such as camomile, cinnamon and garlic.

LIFESTYLE AND ACTIVITIES
- Avoid work or exercise in the hot sun or conditions where your body will become easily overheated
- Avoid mentally stressful activities and situations

MENTAL ATTITUDE
- Avoid anger and grief as much as possible

DRUGS AND THERAPIES
- Detoxification therapy (*shodhana*) – a combination of poorva karma and panchakarma
- Emesis therapy (*vamana*), followed by purgation therapy (*virechana*)
- Enema therapy (*basti*) – both herbal and medicated oil enemas
- Palliative therapy (*shamana*) – herbs with bitter taste, such as vasa (Malabar nut), neem, shatavari

(*Asparagus racemosus Willd.*), amalaki (Indian gooseberry) and kushmanda
- Ayurvedic medicines such as soothashekara ras, shankha bhasma, kamadugha ras or pravala, nimbadi choornam, jeerakadi modaka, pippali ghritam, shatavari ghritam, harikala lavara and bhumimbadi kadha

Prognosis

The symptoms of gastritis are usually relieved within a week, but treatment should be continued for at least three months. Diet and lifestyle changes are necessary to prevent recurrence.

PEPTIC ULCERS

Peptic ulcers are a chronic disorder characterized by frequent recurrences, and which affects one to two per cent of adults. The acid secreted in the stomach and the poor resistance of the mucosal layers of the stomach or duodenum results in peptic ulcers. If the ulcer forms on the wall of the stomach, it is known as a gastric ulcer; if it forms in the duodenum, it is known as a duodenal ulcer.

In ayurvedic medicine, peptic ulcer diseases are commonly categorized under *parinama shoolam* (gastric ulcer) or *annadrava shoolam* (duodenal ulcer). Basically vata dosha, in association with pitta and kapha, manifests symptoms in the stomach which are severe and recurrent.

What causes peptic ulcers?

Excessive use of irritant foods, such as chillies, spices, alcohol, drugs (painkillers and steroids) and stress, can all precipitate an ulcer. The results of recent medical research has shown that the presence of *Helicobacter pylori* in the digestive system is also associated with ulcers. Smoking increases the rate of ulcer recurrence and slows ulcer healing. More rarely, ulceration is also associated with Zollinger-Ellison syndrome, multiple endocrine neoplasia (MEN) syndrome and hyperparathyroidism.

What are the symptoms?

PARINAMA SHOOLA (GASTRIC ULCER)
- Pain in the abdomen which starts immediately after food, but is relieved after the food is completely digested
- Pain is also sometimes felt in the back or lower part of the abdomen

- Pain increases if rice and starchy grains are consumed
- If vata dosha is dominant, you will experience grinding sounds in the stomach, abdominal distension and constipation. Oily substances generally relieve this type of pain
- If the pain is predominantly due to pitta, you will experience thirst, a burning sensation and sweating. Cold substances generally relieve this pain
- If the pain is due to predominant kapha dosha, you will experience vomiting and nausea. Bitter substances generally alleviate this pain

ANNADRAVA SHOOLA (DUODENAL ULCER)

Duodenal ulcer is the most common form of peptic ulcer. It normally presents with a history of periodic epigastric pain. This pain will often wake you during the night (usually between 1 and 3 am), and food, milk and alkalis may relieve it. The symptoms are similar to those of gastric ulcers, but in this case you will generally experience pain regardless of food intake or digestive process.

What is the treatment?

The treatment for peptic ulcers is similar to that used for gastritis (see pages 94–5), except that some emphasis will be given to herbs and herbal medicines with *shulahar* (pain-controlling) and *vatahara* (vata-controlling) actions.

Herbs that have a specific pain-controlling and vata-controlling action include:

- Shatavari (*Asparagus racemosus Willd.*)
- Amalaki (Indian gooseberry)

Shankha bhasma, a type of powdered shell, is also good for relieving pain.

Emesis therapy, purgation therapy and enema therapy, particularly *ksheera basti* (a milk-based enema), are recommended in chronic cases.

Prognosis

Peptic ulcers of recent origin will be cured within two to three weeks, but recurrence is possible. You should follow stringent dietary restrictions and attempt to lead a stress-free life, as far as possible. Your diet should not include spicy and hot food or too much oily food. Remember that milk products are soothing. Also make sure that your stomach is not empty for too long by eating smaller meals more frequently.

INDIGESTION

Indigestion is a common term that covers a variety of symptoms brought on by eating, including heartburn, nausea, flatulence (excessive wind in the stomach or intestine causing belching or discomfort), bloating and abdominal pain. The conventional medical terminology for indigestion is 'dyspepsia'.

What causes indigestion?

Indigestion refers to discomfort in the upper abdomen, often brought on by eating too much and too quickly, or by eating food that is too rich, spicy or fatty. Often, anxiety or stress will lead to nervous indigestion. On occasion, persistent or recurrent indigestion can be associated with a peptic ulcer, oesophagitis (inflammation of the oesophagus) or gallstones.

Even when all the causes listed above are excluded, there still remains a significantly large proportion of the population who complain of persistent indigestion for which no cause can be found. These people are considered to have non-ulcer or functional dyspepsia. It is believed that the symptoms are generated by disturbances in the motor function of the alimentary tract, somewhat similar to the motility disturbances that occur in irritable bowel syndrome. Symptoms of both indigestion and irritable bowel syndrome may be present, suggesting a generalized motility disorder.

Other causes of indigestion

- Alcohol abuse
- Pregnancy
- Psychiatric disorders
- Depressive illness
- Anxiety neurosis

ORGANIC DISEASES OF THE DIGESTIVE SYSTEM
- Pancreatic disease, Crohn's disease, colon cancer

SYSTEMIC DISEASE
- Cardiac, renal (kidney) or hepatic (liver) failure
- Extra-abdominal malignancy such as lung carcinoma

MEDICATION
- NSAIDs (non-steroidal anti-inflammatory drugs)
- Digoxin
- Analgesics
- Antibiotics

Flatulent dyspepsia is often used as a collective term for symptoms, such as early satiety (full feeling in the stomach), flatulence, bloating and belching. These symptoms are almost always the result of functional disorder, sometimes due to Crohn's disease and, occasionally, to biliary disorders.

The ayurvedic view

In ayurveda, indigestion is known as *ajirna*. The theory of digestion is based on the concept of *pachak agni* or pitta (that is, the fire governing digestion, or your digestive juices/enzymes). Deficiency in the quality and quantity of the digestive juices, known as *mandagni* in ayurveda, and deficient digestive juices, are considered responsible for the impairment of digestion, leading to ajirna, or indigestion. Indigestion is classified into five types according to the association of doshas and the type of indigestion:

- *Amajeerna* – due to excessive aggravation of kapha
- *Vishtabdhajeerna* – due to excessive aggravation of vata
- *Vidagadhajeerna* – due to excessive aggravation of pitta
- *Rasaseshajeerna* – food-related indigestion
- *Vishajeerna* – due toxins, for example food poisoning

What are the symptoms?

AMAJEERNA
- Swelling of the face
- A feeling of heaviness in the stomach (early satiety)
- Sour burps or belching
- Nausea

VISHTABDHAJEERNA
- Piercing pain in the abdomen
- Flatulence/bloated feeling
- Constipation
- Belching

VIDAGADHAJEERNA
- Sour burps or belching
- A burning sensation in the chest and abdomen
- Thirst
- Dizziness

RASASESHAJEERNA
- Heaviness in the abdomen and chest
- Bloated feeling in the stomach
- Little or even no desire for food
- Excess saliva in your mouth

VISHAJEERNA
- Sharp pain in the abdomen
- Nausea and vomiting
- Diarrhoea

What is the treatment?

AMAJEERNA
- Fasting is beneficial

VISHTABDHAJEERNA
- Light, easily digestible food is recommended

VIDAGADHAJEERNA
- Emesis therapy (*vamana*)

RASASESHAJEERNA
- Rest
- Herbal medicines to improve digestion

VISHAJEERNA
- Fasting followed by light, easily digestible food until normal digestion is restored

Once your system has been cleansed and lightened, you should keep fasting or remain on a light, easily digestible diet until your strength and the doshas of your body are restored to normal. Appetite stimulants and digestives are administered to restore digestion. The following medicines can be used:

- Bhaskar lavana
- Ajawain
- Ginger and salt
- Chitrakadi vati
- Ashtanga lavana
- Hingvastak churna

SUGGESTED REMEDIES
- A chutney made of fresh mint, dried dates, black pepper, rock salt, fried asafoetida, black resins and cumin seeds with lemon juice is very good for improving your digestive power and appetite.
- Equal quantities of cinnamon, ginger and cardamom ground into a powder are helpful in treating indigestion.
- A mixture of equal parts of green ginger, lemon juice and rock salt, taken before meals, relieves indigestion and improves appetite.

Prognosis

Indigestion usually yields effectively to ayurvedic treatment. It may take about a week until you feel relief, but treatment must be continued for about a month.

Case study: irritable bowel syndrome

Irritable bowel syndrome is a common illness among anxious, tense individuals who tend to either be emotionally insecure or have bad dietary habits, or perhaps both. Sandra Miller was a 35-year-old housewife who had a young child of six and a husband with a busy practice as a solicitor, when she sought ayurvedic treatment for irritable bowel syndrome. Her husband had a practice specializing in marital disputes and many of his clients were women of her age who needed his help during the separation from their husbands.

For almost a year, Sandra had experienced cramp-like pains in her abdomen, at times severe enough to make her wince in pain. She also felt wind and constant gurgling in her intestines, as if water were flowing through them. Bloating after a meal was one of the features of her problem.

These sensations were quite often unrelated to her food intake and occurred whether she had eaten or not. Her family doctor prescribed her a bulk-producing (high-fibre) agent called Fybogel, which did actually help her initially, but Sandra also felt that it sometimes made the cramps worse. She was then asked to undergo a colonoscopy examination which cleared up her diverticulitis.

In the hope of a better solution to her problem, Sandra consulted an ayurvedic physician. The doctor diagnosed her problems as the exacerbation of both vata and pitta, and prescribed a series of panchakarma sessions involving laxatives (virechana) and herbal enemas (basti). She also prescribed the tasty yet powerful vilwadi avaleha (herbal jelly) for the stomach.

The herbal enema completely settled Sandra's stomach cramps and improved her power of digestion. The ayurvedic physician also recommended that she stick to a light, cooked diet, one that was low in fibre (as against the more common recommendation of increasing fibre) and sweet in taste. As Sandra is a high vata-pitta type, the sweet taste is good for her.

It emerged that one of Sandra's main fears was that her husband would leave her for one of his clients. This had made her literally starve herself to avoid putting on weight. Added to this, when she did eat, she usually chose junk food to ease her anxiety, resulting in irritable bowel syndrome. After her treatment, Sandra in fact looked so well and felt so confident that she no longer worried about rivals for her husband's affection.

CONSTIPATION

Constipation is a very common disturbance within the digestive tract which is often seen in developed countries, such as the UK and the USA, where people often have too much processed food in their diet and do not get enough exercise.

This ailment restricts regular bowel movement. Improper stool evacuation produces toxins which find their way into the blood and other systems, and in chronic cases this problem can give rise to serious diseases such as rheumatism, arthritis, haemorrhoids, high blood pressure, migraine and even cancer. Apana vayu (downward-moving air) is out of equilibrium in most cases of constipation.

What causes constipation?

• Improper diet and irregular eating habits
• Insufficient intake of water
• Lack of high-fibre foods, such as whole grains and leafy vegetables in your diet
• Excessive intake of meat
• Irritable colon
• Spastic colon
• Food allergies
• Emotional disturbances
• Lack of physical activity
• Mechanical obstruction to stools

What are its symptoms?

• Infrequent, irregular or difficult bowel movements
• Coated tongue
• Foul breath
• Loss of appetite
• Headaches
• Dizziness
• Dark circles under the eyes
• Depression
• Nausea
• Pimples
• Mouth ulcers
• Diarrhoea alternating with constipation
• Varicose veins
• Pain in the lower abdomen
• Lower back pain
• Acidity and heartburn
• Insomnia

What is the treatment?

DIETARY FACTORS

Foods to eat: broccoli, cereals, dairy products (for example, milk, ghee, cream), green leafy vegetables, spinach, wheat, whole grains and fruits, such as pear, guava, grapes, orange, papaya and figs).

Foods to avoid: cheese, hard-boiled eggs, refined sugar, white flour-based products, such as bread, cakes, pastries, biscuits and cookies.

LIFESTYLE AND ACTIVITIES

- Attend to the call of nature regularly, even if you do not have a motion. however, do not strain or induce urges
- Take regular exercise and brisk walks
- Make sure you sleep well at night

DRUGS AND THERAPIES

- Enema therapy (*basti*)
- Herbs – haritaki (Indian gall nut), ishabgol (*Plantago ispagula*), trivrit, aragwadha and senna leaves (not to be used regularly)
- Ayurvedic herbal formulations – triphala, sukha sarak, choornam, avipathikara choornam and trivritadi leham

Prognosis

The prognosis for curing constipation is usually good, but you may be advised on lifestyle and proper eating habits so that you can avoid this problem recurring or becoming a pattern in your life. You should also be cautioned against the long-term use of laxatives, as they usually only make constipation worse.

DIARRHOEA

The frequent passing of loose or large quantities of stools is called diarrhoea. It is commonly referred to as *atisara* in ayurvedic texts.

As the normal consistency of faecal matter changes, it also takes away with it some of the body's fluids (*rasa*, or plasma) and electrolytes (*kleda*). This can lead to dehydration and possibly other serious conditions.

According to Western medicine, diarrhoea is a symptom, not a disease. It is usually caused by an infection in the intestine, although in some cases it may arise from a more serious systemic condition. Diarrhoea can be extremely dangerous in children, particularly infants or toddlers.

What causes diarrhoea?

- Eating heavy, very fatty or very dry (almost fat-free) foods
- Consuming very hot or very cold meals
- Drinking too much liquid
- Eating too many solids
- Eating incompatible foods (see pages 78–9)
- Eating before the previous meal has been digested or when suffering from indigestion
- Eating an unbalanced diet
- Excessive or improper use of panchakarma (see pages 56–62)
- Poisons or toxins in food
- Psychological causes, such as fear or grief
- Drinking or using impure water
- Excessive wine and alcohol consumption
- Seasonal aberrations
- Too much time spent in the water, for example excessive swimming
- Suppression of natural urges
- Infestation with worms or micro-organisms

There are six types of diarrhoea according to ayurveda:

- Vata diarrhoea
- Pitta/rakta diarrhoea
- Kapha diarrhoea
- Tridosha/sannipaata diarrhoea
- Psychogenic/nervous diarrhoea – diarrhoea caused by fear, grief and stress

For therapeutic purposes, diarrhoea is grouped into two stages: either *ama* diarrhoea or *pakwa* diarrhoea. The type of treatment used varies according to the stage into which it falls. If stools have a very foul odour, are sticky or glue-like, and sink in water, the diarrhoea is at the ama stage. If stools are light and float in water, this indicates the pakwa stage.

There is also another type of diarrhoea known as *rakta* or bloody diarrhoea. This is usually an advanced stage of pitta diarrhoea (excessive pitta is the most common cause of diarrhoea), where the sufferer continues to indulge in consuming excessive pitta-increasing substances, such as chillies, spices or alcohol over a long period of time and the condition deteriorates into rakta diarrhoea.

What are the symptoms?

The different types of diarrhoea produce specific changes in the consistency of your stools, and affect the frequency with which they are passed and associated physical and psychological symptoms.

These changes, which help to diagnose the type of diarrhoa your are suffering, are categorized as follows.

VATA TYPE
- Your stools are reddish or pinkish, frothy, dry, unformed, and contain undigested food
- Small quantities of stool are passed very frequently
- Gas is passed along with the stool

PITTA TYPE
- Your stools are yellowish, bluish and mixed with blood
- You feel very thirsty
- Occasionally, you may faint or feel dizzy
- You experience a burning sensation in the anal region
- The anus sometimes becomes red and inflamed

KAPHA TYPE
- Your stools are whitish, cohesive and sticky, and are cold
- The stools are mixed with mucus and possess a foul smell

TRIDOSHA TYPE
In this type of diarrhoea, you will usually experience a combination of all the symptoms mentioned above. Your stools will be like bacon fat.

NERVOUS DIARRHOEA
Excessive fear or grief impairs vata, which in turn disturbs the functions of the digestive system and damages or weakens the blood vessels. Consequently, your stools become mixed with blood from injured blood vessels in the gut, making the stools reddish in appearance. In nervous diarrhoea, your faeces may or may not have an odour.

What is the treatment?

The treatment of diarrhoea starts with identifying its cause and avoiding it immediately. It is also necessary to know whether the stage of diarrhoea is ama or pakwa, and which type of diarrhoea you are suffering. In the ama stage, no anti-diarrhoeal agents, such as drugs that stop loose stools should be used.

As diarrhoea is an outcome of diminished agni (digestive fire), fasting for a few hours is advisable.

USEFUL HERBS
Recommended for diarrhoea is the use of herbs with *dipaniya* (heat-increasing), *paachana* (digestive) and *stambha* (arresting) properties. These include:

- Ajamoda (*Trachyspernum roxburghianum Sprague.*)
- Amraasthi (inner seed of mango)
- Asafoetida resin (*Ferula foetida Regel.*)
- Ativisha (*Aconitum heterophyllum Wall.*)
- Bilwa (*Aegle marmelos Corr.*)
- Chavya (*Piper chaba Hunter*)
- Chitraka (*Plumbago zeylanica Linn.*)
- Ginger (*Zingiber officinalis Rocs.*)
- Haritaki (*Terminalia chebula Linn.*)
- Kutaja (*Holerrhina antidysenterica Wall.*)
- Lajjalu (*Mimosa pudica Linn.*)
- Lodhra (*Symplocos racemosus Roxb.*)
- Mocharasa (*Salmalia malabarica Schott x Endl.*)
- Pippali (*Piper longum Linn.*)
- Pippalimoola (root of *Piper longum Linn.*)

These herbs can be used as powders, decoctions, fresh juices or as a single-herb drug, but you should always consult an ayurvedic practitioner first. Self-diagnosis and prescription is not recommended.

USEFUL AYURVEDIC MEDICINES
The following ayurvedic medicines are commonly prescribed to treat various forms of diarrhoea. As usual, it is advisable to take these drugs under the supervision of a qualified ayurvedic physician:

- Kutaja ghana vati
- Gangadhara choornam
- Hingwastaka choornam
- Bilwadi choornam
- Kutajarishtam
- Mustakarishtam
- Lashunadi vati
- Snagivim vati
- Pravala panchamrit ras
- Shanka bhasma

WHEN TO STOP TREATMENT?
Treatment for diarrhoea can be stopped when you are able to urinate without passing faeces at the same time, the flatus passes normally and you feel hungry and light in the abdomen.

WHAT FOOD IS RECOMMENDED?
- Boiled water
- Buttermilk
- Rice with meat broth or soup
- Sour gruels, such as tomato soup
- Boiled vegetable soups
- Lemon juice
- Pomegranate juice
- Cooked apples
- Bananas
- Kitchari

Home remedies

USEFUL IN MILD CASES OF DIARRHOEA

- A mixture of equal parts of the tender leaves of the babul tree (*Gum acacia*) with cumin seed and caraway seed, in doses of 12 g each, to be taken three times a day as an infusion.
- Soak 3 g of catechu and a stick of cinnamon in 300 ml (10 fl oz) boiling water for two hours. Allow to cool before using. Take this decoction in 30 ml doses, at room temperature, three times a day.
- Buttermilk by itself is a good home remedy for mild diarrhoea.

Kitchari

Kitchari is also known as kichadi or kitcheri. While the spellings may differ slightly, the principle is always the same. When you need to follow a light, nutritious diet, kitchari is ideal as it is easily digested and is suited to all of the doshas.

The basic recipe is given below, but appropriate vegetables for the season and your dosha can be used if you wish. Root vegetables will need to be added with the rice, while leafy, green vegetables, such as spinach require a shorter cooking time.

> ½ cup split yellow mung beans (moong dal)
> 1 cup basmati rice
> 1–2 tablespoons ghee (clarified butter) or oil
> 2 teaspoons ground cumin
> 2 teaspoons ground coriander
> 2 teaspoons fennel seeds
> 2 teaspoons ground turmeric

Soak the split mung beans in cold water overnight. Rinse thoroughly with fresh cold water at least twice. Mix with the rice and rinse once again.

Heat the ghee or oil in a pan until moderately hot. Add the spices and cook for a minute or two to release the aromas – but do not allow to scorch. Add the rice and bean mixture, stirring gently to coat the grains with the oil and spices.

Now add just enough water to cover the grains by about 5 cm (2 in) and bring to the boil. Cook uncovered for 5 minutes or so. Cover the pan with a lid and simmer gently for 35–40 minutes, or until the rice is cooked. Stir the dish from time to time, and do not allow it to become dry – add extra water as necessary.

The four pillars of treatment

As has been stressed throughout this book, ayurveda does not merely seek to cure disease, but also to restore the equilibrium of the three doshas. It is all about health, wellbeing and a long and happy life.

Part of this philosophy is manifested in the principle of the four pillars of treatment: a good physician, good medication, a good nurse and a good patient.

Of these, a good physician is considered paramount, but the others have important roles as well. Drugs should come from proper sources with proper regard to selection, storage and preparation. The nurse needs to be knowledgeable, skilled, pure in body and mind, and empathetic. And, finally, the patient must have a good memory, be willing to follow instructions, possess courage and be able to describe his or her ailments in an uninhibited manner.

Prognosis

Diarrhoea resulting from disturbances in vata, pitta and kapha is easily treated, and you will get well quickly once you have started treatment, usually within three days. However, tridosha and nervous diarrhoea can be very difficult to treat. Giving an estimate of the time you will need to recover from the latter two conditions is not as clear cut, but your ayurvedic doctor will be able to advise you of the expected prognosis once you are diagnosed and begin treatment. Obviously, in the case of nervous diarrhoea, the added factor of exactly what situations or emotions trigger this condition, and also its chronic nature, will need to be dealt with before you can be free of it.

Caution

If you experience any of the following signs or symptoms when you are suffering from diarrhoea, do not continue ayurvedic treatment. Your ayurvedic physician should immediately refer you to a hospital for specialist care or you should seek this treatment yourself as a matter of urgency:

- If the stools resemble a piece of liver, are very thin, look like oil, fat, bone marrow, milk or yogurt, are black or smell like a cadaver
- If you experience severe thirst, a burning sensation, breathlessness, develop hiccoughs or severe pain in the flanks and bones
- If you develop mental confusion, disorientation, fainting, suppuration of the anus and delirium

Cirrhosis of the liver

The liver is the largest glandular organ in the human body. It performs many vital functions in addition to its main role of producing and excreting bile. These functions include metabolizing carbohydrates, fats and proteins, storing vitamins (A, B12, D, E and K), reproducing haemoglobin, maintaining body temperature, and detoxifying the body of poisonous substances by transforming and removing toxins and wastes. When the liver becomes diseased as a result of infections, drugs, chemicals or alcohol, most of these functions are weakened or lost. Fortunately, the liver has a tremendous capacity to heal itself and correct minor dysfunction.

In ayurveda, the liver is a pitta organ and most of the pitta functions are linked to the functions of the liver. It is also considered as a seat of agni (digestive fire) and the root of the *raktavahasrotas* (the body's channels of the blood). Thus, in liver disease, an abnormality of pitta, agni and rakta (blood) can take place. In ayurveda, most of the liver diseases are treated either as a pitta disease or as a rakta (blood) disease.

Cirrhosis is a disease of the liver caused by chronic damage to the cells. Bands of fibrosis break up the normal structure of the liver. The surviving cells multiply to form regeneration nodules and scar tissue. As these nodules are inadequately supplied with blood, liver function is gradually impaired. The liver no longer effectively removes toxic substances from the blood. In addition, the distortion and fibrosis of the liver leads to portal hypertension. About 4,000 cases of cirrhosis are reported each year in the UK, and approximately 2,500 deaths take place every year as a result of liver failure. In the USA, more than 25,000 people die of liver failure annually.

What causes cirrhosis?

- Heavy alcohol consumption
- Hepatitis – most common in hepatitis B and C
- Rare diseases of the bile duct
- Some drugs
- Haematoma and primary cancer of the liver

What are the symptoms?

Cirrhosis may lead to various complications, any of which may be the first sign of the condition:

- Mental confusion
- Ascites (collection of fluid in the abdominal cavity)
- Aesophageal varices (enlarged vein in the walls of the oesophagus) which can rupture causing vomiting of blood
- Coma

What is the treatment?

Treatment options for the common liver diseases, such as cirrhosis and fatty liver, are problematic in conventional medicine, especially because of the frequent complications that are associated with them.

In recent years, many researchers have examined the effects of plants used traditionally by ayurvedic physicians to support liver function and treat liver diseases. Out of several hundred plants, only a few have been found to be promising and effective for use, as well as safe. They are:

- Katuki (*Picrorrhiza kuroa Benth.*)
- Turmeric (*Curcuma longa Linn.*)
- Liquorice (*Glycyrrhiza glebra Linn.*)
- Punarnava, or red hogweed (*Boerhaavia diffusa Linn.*)

Also, the well-known drug Liv 52 has been shown to have a remarkable effect on cirrhosis of the liver. A number of case studies proving this link are available.

Prognosis

Cirrhosis of the liver is an extremely serious disease. Early treatment by ayurvedic medication can prevent total liver failure provided you live a very careful, moderate lifestyle. It is necessary to avoid alcohol, as well as all of the toxic substances and behaviour that aggravate pitta.

Hepatitis

Among the many diseases that can affect the liver, the most common is hepatitis. Hepatitis can be caused by certain types of medication, viruses, bacteria, some types of mushrooms, parasites such as amoebas or giardia, and liver flukes from dogs or cats. The most common hepatitis viruses affecting the liver are hepatitis A, B, C, D and E.

Hepatitis A is by far the most common form of this disease and is usually transmitted through food and water. Hepatitis A is a self-limiting disease, in most cases lasting for around two weeks, but occasionally it can manifest in a very severe form resulting in liver failure and even death.

Hepatitis B, in contrast, is not so common, but recently there has been a rise in the incidence of this infection. It is usually transmitted through blood, body fluids, serum, saliva, urine and sexual contact. It is also transmitted through breast milk to infants. The medical fraternity is becoming increasingly worried about this chronic type of hepatitis because of its risk of transmission from one person to another, and also because of its association with liver cancer. There is no effective treatment for this type of hepatitis, although a vaccine has been developed as a prophylactic. Its efficacy is doubtful and occasionally the vaccine itself can precipitate the illness.

Hepatitis C is a chronic, fatal infection for which there is no cure or vaccination. Transmission is similar to that of hepatitis B.

Hepatitis E, like hepatitis A, is characterized by oral-faecal transmission. It is also self-limiting in nature.

What are the symptoms?

- Low-grade fever
- Digestive upsets, such as indigestion
- Pain in the abdomen (particularly a tender liver)
- Jaundice (yellow eyes, skin and urine)
- Liver enlargement

According to ayurveda, all these clinical features are usually associated with aggravated pitta. Hence hepatitis is usually diagnosed as a pitta disease or, more precisely, *kaamala* in ayurveda.

What is the treatment?

DIETARY FACTORS
Foods to eat: sweet, cooling foods, fruits and bitter vegetables, such as spinach and Swiss chard, and drink plenty of water

Foods to avoid: alcohol, fats, salt, sour food and fruits including oranges, grapes, yogurt, spices and chillies.

ACTIVITIES AND LIFESTYLE
- Complete bed rest
- Avoid the hot sun and heat in general
- Keep your environment as cool and calm as possible

DRUGS AND THERAPY
- Purification therapy – purgation (*virechana*)
- Herbs and single-drug medicines – bhumyamalaki (*Phyllanthus urinaria Linn.*), bharangaraj (*Eclipta alba Hassk*), katuki (*Picrorrhiza kuroa Benth.*), kumari (aloe vera), bhunimba (*Andrographis peniculata Nees*), punarnava, or red hogweed (*Boerhaavia diffusa Linn.*), vacha (calamus), kirata tikta (*Swertia chirata*)
- Herbal formulations – arogya vardhini, triphala, bhumimbadi kwatha, dhatri louha, narayasa louha

Prognosis

As some types of hepatitis are self-limiting in nature, it is difficult to say how much ayurvedic medicine plays a role in your recovery. However, it will certainly reduce the course of your illness and help you to recover from illness quickly. It will also prevent the development of complications such as liver failure, cirrhosis of the liver or liver cancer.

For chronic forms of hepatitis, such as B and C, ayurvedic herbs will help prevent complications. They can also be used as a prophylactic, as many of these herbs will protect the liver from susceptibility to viruses.

Ayurveda also recommends a stress-free lifestyle and a simple, healthy diet as preventive measures.

Respiratory diseases

The group of organs associated with breathing is known as the respiratory system. Ayurveda refers to this breath of life, or life force, as prana. The name given to the respiratory system, or the group of organs concerned with maintaining life in ayurveda, is *pranavaha srotas*. Human life depends upon respiration, as well as the circulation of blood, digestion of food and activities of our minds and sense organs. Thus, in ayurveda, all the organs concerned with these functions are included under the respiratory system. Manifestations of disease are usually the effect of deranged *pranavaha srotas*.

The organs concerned with respiration are:

- Nose
- Trachea
- Lungs with plurae
- Bronchus
- Chest cage
- Diaphragm

Respiration commences from the first moments of birth and stops only at death. This is a two-phase activity, that is, inspiration or breathing in air, and expiration or breathing out; both of these take place regularly and alternately. Vayu (atmospheric air) enters through your nasal passage, passes down the trachea and into the bronchi, where it fills up the air sacs (alveoli). It is right **WHEN THE RESPIRATORY SYSTEM FAILS, IT PRECIPITATES PROBLEMS FOR THE WHOLE BODY. AYURVEDA RECOGNIZES THE SYMPTOMS IN RELATION TO IMBALANCES IN SPECIFIC DOSHAS**

allowed to stay there for a very short period before being forced out via the same route. This movement of air is brought about by the function of the two subdivisions of vata: *pranavata*, (assisting breathing in) and *udana vata* (assisting breathing out). The respiratory centre, which is the seat of pranavata and is located in the brain, coordinates these two movements.

The passage for breathing is formed out of the mucous membrane, which secretes mucus. This slimy, sticky discharge keeps the air entering the lungs moist and also filters out any foreign material, but if too much mucus is secreted it can cause problems. According to ayurveda, the chest cavity is an important seat of kapha, principally the subdosha of avalambaka kapha.

Blood (*rakta*) is continuously being pumped by the heart into the lungs. The blood exchanges its gaseous wastes, such as carbon dioxide, with oxygen brought in by the atmospheric air. This oxygenation is the main function required for producing heat and energy.

What causes respiratory disease?

Common causes of various respiratory diseases are:

- Exposure to dust, pollen, smoke or cold breezes
- injury
- Exposure to extreme cold
- Excessive physical exertion
- Poisons and toxins
- Suppression of natural urges, such as sneezing, yawning and hiccoughs
- Malnutrition
- Obstruction to the breathing passage
- Infection

What are the symptoms?

Common symptoms of respiratory disease are:

- Running nose
- Nose bleeds
- Obstruction in the throat
- Cough
- Dyspnoea (breathlessness)
- Halitosis (bad breath)
- Chest pain
- Pain in the upper back
- Hoarse voice
- Cyanosis (skin discoloration due to lack of oxygen)

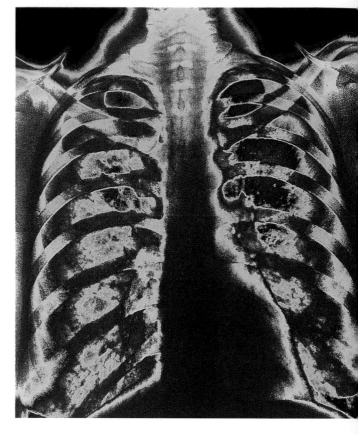

BRONCHITIS

A chronic cough that produces sputum is known as bronchitis. Chronic bronchitis causes about 30,000 deaths per year in the UK and about 55,000 deaths annually in the USA.

Initially, you will develop an acute morning cough and an increased frequency of lower respiratory tract infections, producing infected sputum. Over a period of time, breathing will slowly become more difficult (dyspnoea) and you will start wheezing.

Bronchitis is referred to as *kasa roga* in ayurveda. It is broken down into five types, or categories:

- Vata type
- Pitta type
- Kapha type
- Kshata type (caused by injury to the chest)
- Kshaya type (caused by wasting of tissues or tuberculosis)

Although bronchitis is mainly a kapha imbalance, the other doshas of pitta and vata are also out of equilibrium in this illness.

What causes bronchitis?

- Tobacco smoking
- Atmospheric pollution
- Socioeconomic deprivation – particularly damp, poor-quality housing
- Lowered immunity
- Inadequate clothing and protection for extreme kapha types

What are the symptoms?

VATA TYPE
- Pain in the chest and sides
- Headache
- Hoarse voice
- Dryness in the chest, throat and mouth
- Goose flesh or goose bumps
- Fainting
- Hollow and resonant sound when you cough
- Dry cough
- Sputum is dry and scanty, and there is pain when you cough it up
- Cough aggravated by food and drinks that are unctuous, sour, salty and warm, such as orange juice, buttermilk, yogurt or eggs
- Symptoms worsen after eating, due to upward-moving vayu (air)

PITTA TYPE
- Yellowish sputum
- Yellowish colour of the eyes
- Bitter taste in the mouth
- Impairment of the voice
- Smoky belching
- Thirst
- Burning sensation
- Anorexia
- Dizziness or fainting
- Phlegm mixed with pitta – indicated by colour

KAPHA TYPE
- Loss of appetite
- Vomiting and nausea
- Chronic rhinitis
- Feeling of heaviness in the body
- Goose flesh or goose bumps
- Sweet, sticky sensation in the mouth
- Thick, large quantity of sputum is expectorated
- No pain in the chest region when you cough
- Feeling of fullness in the chest

KSHATA TYPE
This problem usually arises as a result of excessive sexual indulgence, excessive exhaustion, too much walking, running excessively long distances and a general overexertion for an extended period. It is characterized by the following symptoms:

- In the beginning, a dry cough, which will later expectorate sputum along with blood
- Excessive chest pain
- Excessive pain in the throat
- Unable to tolerate touch or your feel pain when touched
- Feeling miserable
- Fever
- Dyspnoea (breathlessness)
- Thirst
- Hoarse voice

KSHAYA TYPE
This form of bronchitis due to pthisis, or tissue wasting, is usually caused due to excessive worry, unwholesome food, an immensely hateful disposition, overindulgence in sex or suppression of natural urges. It presents with the following symptoms:

- Coughing out sputum that is foul smelling, green or red in colour and may appear like pus
- Desire for large quantity of food
- Weakness and emaciation
- Face, complexion and skin becoming pale and unctuous
- Soles of the feet and palms of the hand becoming smooth and shiny
- A hateful disposition and always trying to find fault with others
- Fever
- Chronic rhinitis
- Anorexia
- Pain in chest region and sides of the chest
- Stools are sometimes hard and at other times loose, without any obvious cause
- Hoarse voice

What is the treatment?

It is very important to avoid all causative factors for bronchitis as far as possible.

VATA TYPE
In vata-type bronchitis, if you are suffering from constipation and flatulence, treatment consists of enemas (basti). If you have dryness of the chest and symptoms of a kapha imbalance, the first step is purgation therapy (virechana) with the following drugs:

- Vasa (Malabar nut)
- Kantakari (Solanum xanthocarpum)

- Kantakari ghritham
- Agastya haritaki
- Stipoladi choornam

PITTA TYPE
In pitta-type bronchitis, if you show signs of aggravated kapha, emesis therapy (*vamana*) is carried out first. After this, you will be given cooling therapy. If the sputum is very thin, then purgation therapy (*virechana*) is administered first. The following herbal medicines are useful:

- Sarkaradi leham
- Pippalyadi leham
- Vidaryadi kashayam
- Drakshadi kashayam

KAPHA TYPE
In kapha-type bronchitis, if you are basically strong, emesis therapy (*vamana*) is done first, followed by medicated smoking (*dhooma*). You may be advised to drink honey, sour drinks such as orange juice, warm water, buttermilk or low alcohol drinks.

The following herbal medicines are useful:

- Dashamoola haritaki kashayam
- Dashamoolarishtam
- Vasakaristam
- Dasamooladi ghritham
- Dasamoola haritaki leham

KSHATA AND KSHAYA TYPES
Bronchitis of kshata and kshaya types is treated in the same way as vata-type bronchitis, but great care should be taken to provide rest, proper nutrition and psychological support, as well as medication.

Prognosis

Bronchitis caused by aggravated vata, pitta or kapha, is usually cured after 10–15 days of treatment. The other two types of bronchitis, kshata and kshaya, are difficult to cure, but symptomatic relief is possible.

BRONCHIAL ASTHMA

Asthma is characterized by recurrent shortness of breath, wheezing or coughing caused by reversible narrowing of the airway lumen. The principal cause of increased airway resistance is narrowing of the smooth muscles of the windpipe as a result of hypersensitivity to many different stimuli, such as cold air, dust, or as a result of exercise, emotional distress or allergies.

Thickening of the airways by swelling, as well as blockages of the airway by mucus and secretions, also contributes to asthma. Wheezing is not an essential feature. Asthma is sometimes classified into extrinsic and intrinsic, although treatment for both types is the same. Asthma affects about five to seven per cent of the population of Europe and four to six per cent of population of the USA.

Clinically, asthma manifests as either an acute or a recurrent attack. An acute asthmatic attack is fairly abrupt in onset and is either only a few hours in duration, or spread over a longer period of a week or two. Longer severe attacks are called status astermaticus. If you suffer from asthma, you will feel a tightness in your chest and both inhalation and exhalation become difficult. There may be a cough, which is initially dry, but later produces sputum. Someone suffering from an asthma attack usually sits up with an overinflated chest and has an audible expiratory wheeze. Acute attacks are precipitated by specific allergies caused by such things as pollens or house dust mites, exertion, excitement, cold air or some drugs.

Case study: asthma

Emma Jenkins is a schoolteacher of 40. From the age of 30, she began having regular asthma attacks, initially only in the winter months. Her asthma progressively worsened until she experienced attacks all year round. Her doctor prescribed Salbutamol tablets and then Ventolin inhalers as the attacks worsened. Finally, he gave her Becotide inhalers, which contain corticosteroids to lessen the inflammation in the bronchial tubes.

Emma came to the Ayurvedic Hospital in the hope of being able to discard the inhalers. She was immediately put onto a combination of yoga and medication, as well as shirodhara (see page 64).

Yogic breathing (*pranayama*) brought about an immediate improvement in Emma's breathing. Her ayurvedic medication included chyavanprash (a sweetish jam-like concoction made from gooseberries) and pravala bhasma (a powdery substance derived from coral). Within two weeks, her breathing improved still further.

She is now completely off the inhalers and recently went on a hike through the Welsh hills – something which she could never have attempted before.

Many people suffer recurrent on and off attacks with coughing, wheezing, breathlessness and tightness in the chest, alternating with periods apparently unrestricted, breathing. Intrinsic and emotional factors must be considered simultaneously with allergies.

The ayurvedic diagnosis of asthma is *takamak swasa*. It is basically a condition where kapha and vata are unbalanced, which has its origin in pittasthana.

What causes bronchial asthma?

- Exercise and intake of food which is heavy and unctuous, such as oily and fried foods
- Foods which assist the movement of wind in the stomach, as well as those which obstruct the channels of circulation
- Cold food and drinks
- Dust, smoke and pollens
- Overexertion
- Heavy lifting
- Suppression of natural urges, such as sneezing

How does the disease develop?

The causes of asthma corrupt the vayu (air) moving upwards (*udana vata*) and aggravate kapha. This produces stiffness in the neck and head, leading to the development of rhinitis. The aggravated doshas further obstruct the free movement of air through the air passages, causing shortness of breath and wheezing.

What are the symptoms?

- Breathing becomes very fast and laboured
- Coughing
- Wheezing
- If no phlegm is produced when coughing, the person becomes exceedingly miserable. Expectoration does bring some relief
- Speech is possible only with great discomfort
- It is difficult to lie down on a bed. As a result, a person suffering an asthma attack commonly prefers to sit upright
- Desire for hot things
- Symptoms come in waves followed by an attack-free period
- Symptoms are aggravated by atmospheric conditions, such as cloud, rain, cold and wind

What is the treatment?

In the cases of acute severe asthma attacks, you are advised to seek emergency treatment from your local hospital immediately.

Ayurvedic treatments are beneficial in the case of mild asthmatic symptoms and to prevent the onset of an acute attack. If you suffer from asthma, it is important first to avoid all causative and aggravating factors (triggers) which contribute to your condition.

DIETARY FACTORS
Foods to eat: ginger tea, hot water, jaggery and mustard oil linctus.

Foods to avoid: alcohol, artificial preservatives, additives and colouring agents, black gram, cold or frozen food and drinks, fish, heavy food, milk, oily and fried foods.

LIFESTYLE AND ACTIVITIES
- Ensure your home has proper ventilation and is free from environmental pollution
- Avoid overexercising
- Avoid smoking
- Dress appropriately to protect yourself from cold air and avoid getting wet in the rain or snow

DRUGS AND THERAPY
- Massage over chest and back with warm oil mixed with salt
- Sweating therapy (*swedana*)
- Emesis therapy (*vamana*)
- Purgation therapy (*virechana*)
- Herbal gargles
- Herbal smoking
- Herbs – pippali (*Piper longum Linn.*), turmeric (*Curcuma longa Linn.*), vasa (Malabar nut), kantakari (*Solanum xanthocarpum*), liquorice (*Glycyzrrhisa glabra Linn.*)
- Herbal formulations – vasavalcham, pippalyasavam, haridra bhanda, chyavanprash, kanakasavam, swaskuta ras, vardhamana pippali rasayana, talisapatradi choornam, dashamoola katutraya kashayam, sivasa dasa chintamaki ras

Prognosis

These days asthma is not generally a life-threatening disease. However, chronic asthma and the heavy use of steroids and other inhalers, a sedentary lifestyle and an inappropriate diet over a period of time, can create a situation where delayed treatment for an acute attack can lead to death.

Adopting an suitable lifestyle with light food, warm clothing, regular exercise, yoga, yogic breathing (*pranayama*) and ayurvedic medicine, can control or make asthma a more manageable disease, if not cure it. Even many difficult cases can be cured completely.

ALLERGIC RHINITIS

Inflammation of the mucous membrane that lines the nose due to allergy to pollen, dust or other airborne substances, is known as allergic rhinitis, commonly called hay fever. This ailment can make a sufferer feel miserable while it lasts, particularly if the triggers for it – such as pollen or dust – cannot be avoided completely. In fact, this option is often far too restrictive and impractical to achieve.

Allergic rhinitis can be seasonal or perennial, depending on the type of allergy you have. It is usually manifested by some combination of a blocked nose, nasal discharge, sneezing and facial pressure or pain. Various types of rhinitis are frequently encountered in general medical practice, such as viral, allergic, vaso-motor, hypertrophic and atrophic. Viral and allergic rhinitis are the most common.

What causes allergic rhinitis?

Allergic rhinitis (hay fever) has a wide range of possible triggers depending on the particular allergy or sensitivity from which you suffer. Among the most common are:

- Pollen
- Dust
- Perfume
- Chemical detergents
- Cats and dogs

What are the symptoms?

- Sneezing
- Running nose
- Blocked nose or nasal congestion
- Pain or pressure in the sinuses
- General body ache
- Itchy or burning eyes

Ayurvedic science describes various diseases related to the nose. *Peenasa kshavathu* is similar to the disease known as allergic rhinitis in Western medicine. Basically, people who have allergies to certain things show signs of chronic sluggish digestive fire (*agnimandya*), as a result of which ama (toxins) build up in the system. Ama results in poor quality of tissues and a sluggish immune system. Kapha dosha, which is also responsible for natural resistance, becomes aggravated in this condition and gives rise to the symptoms of allergic rhinitis.

What is the treatment?

If your agni (digestive fire) is dull, then digestive and carminative herbs such as ginger, black pepper, coriander and trikatu – a blend of pippali (*Piper longum Linn.*), black pepper and ginger – should be used initially to strengthen your agni. This will also digest any ama. Once ama is removed, you may be given panchakarma, such as emesis therapy (*vamana*), nasal therapy (*nasya*) and medicated smoking (*dhooma*) to clear excess doshas from your body. When properly purified, you should receive rejuvenation therapy (*rasayana*) for between five and six months.

The best forms of rejuvenation therapy will be with the following ayurvedic medicines:

- Chyavanprash
- Vardhaman pippali rasayan
- Brahma rasayan
- Haridra khanda
- Vyoshadi vatakam

Prognosis

The prognosis for allergic rhinitis depends very much on you as an individual and your immune system. Generally, ayurvedic treatment over a period of five to six months should help hay-fever sufferers to develop proper resistance. Seasonal purification as advised in ayurvedic medicine (see pages 70–71) and undergoing rejuvenation therapy (page 86) just before the expected season of hay fever is also recommended.

SINUSITIS

Sinusitis refers to an inflammation of the mucous membrane lining the paranasal sinuses. It is often a result of a common cold, influenza or other general infections. Germs sometimes find their way into the sinuses on either side of the nasal passage, leading to health problems. In ayurveda, sinusitis is diagnosed as *shirashool*, which in most instances is the result of a kapha imbalance.

What causes sinusitis?

- Allergic rhinitis (hay fever)
- Deviated nasal septum
- Excessive kapha
- Poor dental hygiene
- Overindulgence in chocolate, yogurt and other kapha-producing foods
- Untreated colds

What are the symptoms?

A recurrent common cold is the first stage of this disease, followed by the symptoms below:

- Excessive or constant sneezing
- Running nose
- Blocked nostrils
- Headache usually felt in the forehead and just below the eyes – aggravated by movement and bending forwards
- Low-grade fever
- Lack of appetite
- Difficulty in breathing
- Heaviness in the head

What is the treatment?

DIETARY FACTORS
Foods to eat: light food, warm food that is not oily, warm teas to sip.

Foods to avoid: all fruits and sweets, dairy products, frozen foods, oily fried foods.

LIFESTYLE AND ACTIVITIES
- Keep indoors as much as possible
- Cover your head with a scarf or hat
- Avoid washing your hair
- Do not expose yourself to cold and dust
- Protect yourself from getting wet in the rain

DRUGS AND THERAPIES
- Detoxification therapy (*shodhana* – a combination of poorva karma and panchakarma)
- Emesis therapy (*vamana*)
- Nasal instillation (*nasya*) of medicated oils such as anu taila and shadbindu taila
- Warm herbal paste (*lepa*) made with rasnadi choornam on the forehead and scalp
- Herbs (restorative) – basil or holy basil (*Ocimum* spp.), vasa (Malabar nut), turmeric, ginger, pippalimoola (root of *Piper longum Linn.*)
- Herbal formulations – shirah shooladi vajra ras, laxmi vilas ras, godanti bhasma, mrityunlaya ras

Home remedies

- Freshly grated ginger and a teaspoon of honey can help to clear congested sinuses. You can take this two or three times a day, as required
- Include coriander, basil, turmeric and ginger in your diet. Basil and ginger tea are useful
- Practise yoga and breathing techniques

STEAM INHALATIONS
Steam inhalations also help to clear congestion. You could try the following remedies if your sinuses are blocked. Simply pour boiling water into a bowl, lean over the bowl carefully and inhale deeply. Make sure that you keep your head covered with a towel while inhaling, so that you retain as much of the steam as possible and you gain the full benefit.

- Add 1 teaspoon eucalyptus oil to a bowl of boiling water and inhale
- Boil about 4 tablespoons of coriander seed along with the water. Transfer to a bowl and inhale
- Boil some freshly chopped ginger (a piece about 1 cm/½ in long) with water. Transfer to a bowl and inhale. Fresh ginger is best, but you can use ground ginger if you do not have any

Prognosis

Sinusitus responds quite well to ayurvedic treatment. Once the initial infection has been cleared, you can incorporate preventive measures into your daily lifestyle, such as avoiding dairy products, cold drinks and smoking, to ensure it does not become chronic.

Migraine

Migraine, if you will pardon the pun, can be a real headache for the physician to treat successfully. Nowadays, this extremely painful type of headache is becoming a more common problem because of our increasingly busy lives and the subsequent stress this places on our bodies and our minds.

If you suffer from frequent and persistent migraines, it is important that you have a complete medical evaluation by an ayurvedic physician, including a thorough look at your history to identify personal or environmental factors that may trigger your attacks.

According to ayurveda, migraine is caused by vata dosha and can be compared with *ardha vabhedhaba*, a one-sided headache that occurs mainly in mentally vulnerable people and those with a vata constitution. It is predominantly the result of aggravated pitta, but can also result from a vata or a kapha imbalance.

What causes migraine?

- Dry food
- Lack of sleep
- Overwork or stress
- Exposure to extreme hot and cold

- Muscular tension
- Hormonal contraceptives
- Hormonal fluctuation in menstrual cycle
- Antihypertensive agents
- Food triggers, such as cheese and alcohol

What are the symptoms?

- Headache which is often limited to one side
- Extreme sensitivity to light or sound
- Pain exacerbated by movement
- Visual disturbances, such as spots or flashes of light before the eyes
- Sometimes accompanied by nausea and vomiting
- Loss of appetite
- Symptoms worsened by emotions and fasting

What is the treatment?

- Nasal therapy (nasya) – administration of medicine through the nose
- Shirodhara
- Guggulu (Commiphora mukul)
- Rasna (galangal)
- Eranda (castor oil plant)

Prognosis

Treatment for migraine in ayurveda is highly effective. In recent years, scientific studies have been done to evaluate the efficacy of ayurvedic treatment for this ailment. The herbs and therapies listed above have been shown to have a significant effect on alleviating migraine, regardless of frequency or severity.

Gynaecological disorders

The authentic texts of ayurveda have all discussed the subject of obstetrics and gynaecology in various sections. Anatomy and physiology have been dealt with in detail in the *Sarir Sthana*. Other sections – apart from those concerning anatomy and physiology – also deal with the various diseases and the treatment involved. Many of the diseases we know today are not mentioned as independent diseases, but rather are present as a subtype or a feature of another disease. For example, the broad category of *yoni vyapat* (disorders of the yoni) resembles conditions such as endometriosis, dysmenorrhoea, presacral neuralgia and cribriform hymen.

Case study: migraine

Richard Simkin suffered from acute migraine for several years. As an investment banker, he could not afford to miss work, so he suffered through painful migraine attacks by taking powerful painkillers, which also upset his stomach. Eventually, he developed a stomach ulcer and the doctor advised him to cut down on the painkillers. This meant he had to stay at home when he had a migraine, as it was impossible to work with the pain.

In desperation, he called the Ayurvedic Hospital, as he had heard that ayurveda cured migraine. He was examined by an ayurvedic doctor, who diagnosed him as having a kapha-vata constitution. He was also told that he had a deviated nasal septum (where the cartilage between the nostrils is bent to one side).

The doctor advised nasal therapy in the form of nasal drops for a 16-day period, combined with guggul as internal medication, as well as an oil to massage on his head. The nasal drops brought out a great deal of accumulated phlegm from the sinuses and the oil had a soothing effect. Within one month of treatment, Richard's migraines had disappeared completely and have not since returned.

MENORRHAGIA

Abnormal bleeding (haemorrhage) from the uterus and vagina is quite a common complaint among menstruating women. It can be of various types:

- Increased amount
- Increased duration
- Shortened interval
- Irregular bleeding

In ayurveda, this type of abnormal bleeding is known as:

- *Rajovridhi*
- *Artaravriddhi*
- *Raktapradar* or *asrigdara*

Menorrhagia is excessive menstrual bleeding. It is usually associated with aggravated pitta.

What causes menorrhagia?

- Endometriosis
- Polycystic ovarian syndrome
- Polyps and tumours

- Unresolved anger or resentment
- Too much hot, spicy, sour or salty food
- Smoking and alcohol

What are the symptoms?

- Excessive bleeding via the vagina
- General body aches and pains
- Possible dizziness and fainting
- Pallor
- Thirst

What is the treatment?

- Adequate rest
- Liquid nutritious diet
- Cold compress on the lower abdomen
- Vaginal douches (*uttara basti*) – panchavalkala decoction, saurashtri jala (alum), triphala decoction
- Ayurvedic medicines – pushyanuga choornam, pradarantaka rasa, shatavari ghrita, asokarishta, pradarari loha, kushamanda khanda, ashoka ghrita, lodhrasava

Prognosis

Treating the pain and discomfort of menorrhagia can be very effective, once any serious underlying cause has been ruled out. Once again it is crucial to adopt a strategy to prevent menstrual problems. Yoga, aloe vera gel and following a diet suitable for your individual constitution can be extremely helpful in this.

ENDOMETRIOSIS

Endometriosis, where during the menstrual cycle tissue from the uterine lining attaches itself to other body organs, is known as *vataja yonivyapat* in ayurveda.

What causes endometriosis?

Endometriosis is an imbalance of vata dosha – as a result of vata-increasing diet and activities – leading to aggravated vata in the genital tract, which becomes dry and rough as a result of this imbalance.

What are the symptoms?

- Painful periods
- Menstrual bleeding other than from the vagina, for example rectal bleeding
- Tingling sensation in the vagina
- Pain in the groin and flanks
- Lower back pain

What is the treatment?

- Oil therapy (*snehana*)
- Sweating therapy (*swedana*) – usna sweda on the lower abdomen
- Detoxification therapy (*shodhana*) – a combination of poorva karma and panchakarma
- Massage and herbal enemas
- Nutritious diet
- Vaginal douches – decoction of fanti, triphala and guduci; decoction of dashamoola
- Tampons – medicated oil of guduci, rasna, bala, chitrak and devadaru; medicated oil of saindhava, kushtha, brhati and devadaru; narayan taila
- Ayurvedic medicines – bolbadha rasa, kumarika (aloe vera) vati, rajahpravartini vati, bhallatakavleha

Prognosis

Endometriosis is sometimes treated by surgery in Western medicine, but again ayurveda can effectively treat this condition, particularly with the use of aloe vera in either gel or tablet form.

PREMENSTRUAL SYNDROME

Menstruation is a natural part of life. It is God's gift to the living beings of the universe to maintain health by eliminating toxic material from the body. Natural detoxification or elimination of toxic material in the form of menstrual blood is a health-preserving gift to women so that generations can be maintained and continued.

Premenstrual syndrome (PMS), which is also known as premenstrual tension (PMT), is characterized by pain, discomfort and symptoms before menstruation. It occurs because of vata dosha and some functional impairment in the *arthavahasrotas* (channels carrying menstrual fluid) of the female reproductive system.

Approximately 50–75 per cent of women suffer from PMS, and it is most likely to occur between the ages of 20 and 30 years. So far, how exactly PMS occurs is not clearly understood. A wide variety of symptoms can be present, and many women learn to recognize these and use them as a signal of when menstruation is about to start.

What causes PMS?

- Irregular diet
- Mutually contradicting food

- Emotion
- Unhealthy sexual practice
- Lack of nourishment
- Psychological and family problems
- Problems with sexual partners

What are the symptoms?

- Pain and swelling in the breasts
- Salt and sweet cravings
- Loss of sleep
- Mental confusion
- Headache
- Anxiety and depression
- Abdominal pain and bloating
- Palpitation

What is the treatment?

- Purgation therapy (*virechana*)
- Enema therapy (*basti*)
- Ayurvedic medicines – pushyanuga choornam, rajapravrattini vati

Prognosis

Ayurveda can give relief to or cure women suffering PMS through its holistic measures.

Skin diseases

According to ayurveda, there are seven subtissues (*upadhatus*) that are evolved out of the body's tissues (*dhatus*), and the skin, or *tvak*, is one of these. It is described in detail in the classic ayurvedic texts with all its layers and functions. The seven layers of skin, as discussed in *Sushruta Samhita*, are:

- *Avabhasini* (the top layer of skin)
- *Lohita*
- *Sveta*
- *Tamra*
- *Vedini*
- *Rohini*
- *Mansa dhara* (subcutaneous tissue)

All these layers are described with their normal thickness and functions, and the subsequent disorders involving each layer. For example, the second fold of skin, lohita, is the site for pigmentation changes.

In ayurvedic texts, *kushta* is a term used to indicate skin disorders, although some other minor skin diseases are given in other sections. A number of

precautionary methods are mentioned to keep the skin healthy, glowing and free from disorders. The following oils (pure or medicated with herbs) are used to treat skin disorders:

- Mustard oil (pure or with turmeric)
- Sesame oil
- Olive oil
- Coconut oil
- Neem oil (margosa)
- Sandalwood oil

The main preventive treatment is to keep your skin hygienically clean and regular apply soothing oils and pastes to improve its condition.

ECZEMA

Eczema and dermatitis are characterized by subtle and numerous eruptions with exudation itching and a burning sensation. The rashes can sometimes also be dry, but itching is the most important sign.

What is the treatment?

The first line of treatment in ayurveda is to relieve the itching by the application of soothing ointments or oils. Once the itching is relieved, the eruptions begin to heal quickly.

EXTERNAL APPLICATION
- Neem oil
- Mahamaricadi oil
- Kasisadi ghrta
- Karanja oil (oil from the seeds of *Pongamia pinnata*)

INTERNAL USE
- Mahamanjisthadi Kvath
- Sarivadyarishta
- Gandhak rasayana

VITILIGO

Vitiligo (*svitra*), also known as Leukoderma, is a disease of the skin characterized by white, light red or coppery patches caused by a loss of pigmentation. This skin condition is caused by the vitiation of all three doshas and is curable if:

- The hair over the patches has not turned white
- The patches (white or coppery) are not numerous
- The patches are of recent origin
- They are not the result of a burn

What is the treatment?

Despite of its non-infective nature, vitiligo can cause considerable emotional suffering for those people affected by it. The following drugs are recommended for treating the condition:

- Bakuchi (*Psorelia corylifolia*) – for both local and oral use
- Gunjadi taila – for local application

ALOPECIA

In ayurveda, *indralupta* is the term used to define alopecia or baldness. Damaged vata afflicts the pitta located at the root of the hair shaft and this causes hair depletion; a further blockage by kapha and blood or the hair follicles themselves prevents any new growth of hair.

What is the treatment?

- Paste of the seeds of gunja (*Abrus precatoris*) applied to the scalp
- Application of the juice of brahmi (gotu kola) mixed with honey
- Head massage using bhringaraja oil
- Paste of black pepper rubbed onto the scalp to encourage growth of new hair
- Rejuvenating (rasyana) drugs

PSORIASIS

In ayurveda, *vicharchika* is the skin disease that most closely resembles the condition known as psoriasis, where there are well-defined patches of red skin. These vary in size from very small patches to much larger areas and can occur on any part of the body, but they appear more commonly on the knees and elbows. When the scales are scraped, they produce a shiny, silvery surface, which is an obvious diagnostic feature.

What is the treatment?

EXTERNAL APPLICATION
- Karanja taila
- Sidhmar kilasa hara taila

INTERNAL USE
- Panchatikta ghrta guggulu
- Mahamanjisthadi kashayam
- Gandhak rasana

Urinary disorders

In ayurveda, the urinary system is referred to as the *mootravahasrota* and includes the kidneys, ureters, bladder and urethra. The kidneys are seen as the head of the urinary system and are connected to the bladder through the ureters. The opening of the bladder extends to the urethra, the passage through which urine is expelled via the external urethral meatus.

Urine is the liquid waste product of the body. It is formed in the kidneys by thousands of small units which secrete urine; through the ureters, it is carried to the bladder for storage and excretion. Rasa (body fluids), together with water and soluble waste products absorbed from the intestine, goes into circulation, supplying nutrition to all the tissues and carrying waste products from the tissues in return. The liquid waste products reach the kidneys and skin for their excretion. Our urinary system has a capacity of about 600 ml (20 fl oz).

The expulsion of urine, which includes contraction of the bladder and relaxation of the sphincter, is controlled by saman vayu and apana vayu, two of the subtypes of vayu (air). The basic elements of water and earth are predominant in urine itself.

Functions of the urinary system

- Regulation of the water content of the body
- Excretion of waste metabolic products
- Retention of substances vital to the body
- Regulation of the electrolyte balance of the body
- Maintenance of the normal acidic balance of the body's fluids

What causes urinary disease?

- Frequent suppression of the urge to urinate
- Low fluid intake
- Extreme exhaustion
- Injury to a part of the urinary system
- Overindulgence in the sexual act

What are the symptoms?

- Polyuria (excessive urine output)
- Dysuria (low urine output)
- Retention of urine
- Urinary incontinence
- Pain in the bladder or kidney region
- Haematuria (blood or red blood cells in the urine)

FEATURES OF INCREASED URINATION
- Distension and pain in the bladder
- Frequent urge to pass urine
- Feeling of a full bladder, even after passing urine

FEATURES OF LOW URINE OUTPUT
- Dysuria (scanty urination)
- Pain in the bladder
- Dark-coloured or bloodstained urine
- Thirst and dryness of the mouth

FEATURES OF URINARY CALCIFICATION
Urinary calcification is known as *ashmari* in ayurveda. In this context, it refers to urinary calculi, or stones. The basic element earth and kapha dosha are both dominant in calculi. The features are:

- Colicky pain in the region of the kidneys, bladder, glans, penis or perineum
- Urine of differing colours depending on the dominant dosha
- Disturbed urinary flow if the stone obstructs the passage (urethra)
- Blood in the urine (haematuria) if the stone causes ulceration of the urinary lining
- Passing of gravel or small particles of stone

Other urinary system disorders include renal colic, haematuria, tumours of the urinary tract and renal failure. Conditions such as hypertension (high blood pressure) are also associated with the urinary system.

What is the treatment?

Urinary disorders are treated by a combination of herbal medicine, panchakarma and diet, including:

- Ayurvedic medication – varunadi kashayam, gokshuradi guggulu, vanga bhasma, praval bhasma, shilajit, punarvasa
- Uttara vasti – enema into the urethra and vaginal passages to help heal the inflammation in the urethra, bladder and the prostate

Diet and lifestyle changes are an important part of the treatment for urinary disorders. During treatment, sexual activity is completely prohibited. You should also avoid coffee, alcohol, spicy food, meat, cold draughts, cold weather, cold baths and horse riding.

CYSTITIS

Cystitis is a very common complaint which largely affects women. A great many women aged between 15 and 35 suffer from painful urination and sometimes bleeding from the urethra. Cystitis rarely affects men, but when it does, it can potentially have more serious consequences than it does for women. This ailment is more common in women because the female urethra is shorter and is more prone to infection as it is closer to ano-rectal region.

What causes cystitis?

Cystitis is caused by aggravated vata or pitta through:

- Excessive spicy foods
- Excessive wine and beer
- Cold weather
- Unhygienic sex
- Lack of cleanliness after sexual activity
- Using toilet paper in the wrong direction (contaminating the urethra with faecal matter)

Case study: cystitis

Pippa Turnbull (29) was subject to frequent attacks of cystitis. She reached the point where she was suffering an attack every two months, often after sex with her boyfriend. Each time she had a bout of cystitis, she was prescribed the antibiotic Bactrim by her GP, which left her feeling nauseous and debilitated at the end of each attack, even though it immediately eased the pain.

In an effort to avoid such a reliance on antibiotics and also to overcome her chronic symptoms, she sought help from the ayurvedic specialist at the Ayurvedic Charitable Hospital. Here she was diagnosed as a vata-pitta type and the following medication was suggested: cystese (containing the herb gokshur), chandansavam (containing sandalwood) and satavarigulam (containing *Asparagus racemosus*)

Within two days, the pain had eased and, after only another two months of treatment, Pippa was completely clear of the symptoms of cystitis. She has remained free of this problem ever since. As part of her continuing treatment, she was also asked to:

- Keep warm in winter, particularly her pelvic area
- Clean her vaginal areas thoroughly after sex
- Keep very strict personal hygiene
- Always ensure she wiped toilet paper away from the direction of her vagina after defecation
- Avoid beer, coffee and white wine
- Avoid spicy food

Case study: erectile dysfunction and premature ejaculation

Len Simmonds, at 45, was a strapping male with a strong, athletic physique and a healthy lifestyle. However, Len, who was popular with women, had a complaint that made him lonely and dejected. Despite his attractiveness to women, after his divorce from his first wife five years before, he had become unable to maintain a satisfactory erection. He even suspected that it had been his inability to satisfy his wife's sexual needs that had made her have the extramarital affairs that broke his heart.

Len decided to consult an ayurvedic physician, who saw Len as having extremely low self-esteem and a wounded soul, which could only be repaired by yogic exercise and meditation to clear his mind. The physician also carried out an astrological analysis of Len's chart, which showed that the split with his wife was due to mutual incompatibility and not sexual dissatisfaction. To improve Len's libido and sexual performance, he prescribed Prolong tablets and Potentex, an oil that includes more than 50 herbs, to rub on his penis.

Within 2 months, Len's erection and premature ejaculation problems had disappeared completely, and he felt that he was able to give satisfactory pleasure to his new-found love.

What are the symptoms?

- Burning sensation when urinating
- Frequent urge to urinate
- Difficulty urinating
- Inflammation of the bladder and urethra

What is the treatment?

Treatment for cystitis is similar to that for other urinary disorders, that is, a combination of herbal medicine, panchakarma, diet and lifestyle changes. It is very important that you adhere to strict personal hygiene and that you avoid aggravating factors such as coffee, carbonated drinks and alcohol.

HOME REMEDY
Coriander seed is helpful for restoring the alkaline balance in your urine and easing any burning sensation. Simply boil 4 tablespoons of coriander seed in 4 cups (2 pints) water until the volume is reduced by half. Drink this solution every day for a week.

Male sexual problems

Healthy sex is a natural part of life, as its basic aim is to produce progeny. If the sexual process is disturbed, it causes other disorders. A sexual problem that affects either male or female, or both, can cause great distress to both partners. In many cases, communication is hampered. It also affects family members as a result of the tension between partners.

All men experience sexual difficulties at one time or another. These problems, particularly dysfunction in males, may cause great anxiety and mental anguish because the sexual act is strongly connected with the image of masculinity. Yet, premature ejaculation, erectile dysfunction, late ejaculation and lack of sexual desire, are quite common.

Ayurveda explains male sexual dysfunction in detail. It is caused by all three doshas and mainly by apana vayu (downward moving air), which makes it difficult to perform satisfactory sex. Sexual dysfunction also occurs because of vitiation of the *shukravahasrotas* (body channels supplying reproductive tissue) of the male reproductive system.

What causes male sexual problems?

- Psychological disorders
- Physical disorders
- Lack of confidence
- Defect in the reproductive system
- Arteriosclerosis (hardening of the arteries)

What are the symptoms?

- Erectile dysfunction – failure to have or maintain an erection, or to penetrate
- Premature ejaculation
- Retorted (delayed) ejaculation
- Lack of sexual desire

What is the treatment?

Recent research has found that some very strong drugs such as Viagra have potentially life-threatening side effects. Ayurveda effectively treats male sexual problems with the following therapies and medicines:

- Detoxification therapy – panchakarma
- Ashwagandha (Withania somnifera)
- Kapikachhu (Mucusa protritis)
- Masha (black gram)
- Shilajatu

Mental illnesses

In ayurveda, the functions of the manas, or mind, are the control of the sense organs and control of the mind itself. In a broader sense, it is responsible for:

- *Cintana* (thinking)
- *Vicara* (consideration)
- *Uha* (speculation)
- *Dhyana* (concentration)
- *Sankalpa* (determination)
- *Indriya graha* (control of senses)
- *Svanigraha* (self-control)

Ayurveda categorizes the causes of mental illness as:

- *Pragyaparadha* (intellectual blasphemy)
- A*satmyendriyartha samyoga* (unwholesome contact of sense organs with their objects)
- *Parinama* (seasonal variation)

Pragyaparadha is considered of prime importance, as Charaka states that a person whose intellect, willpower and memory are deranged indulges in undesired acts, resulting in various disorders. *Asatmyendriyartha samyoga* and *parinama* also bring about different kinds of diseases of the body and mind. Hence ayurveda's psychosomatic approach to treatment. In the words of Rena Dubos: 'Whatever its precipitating cause and its manifestations, almost every disease involves both body and mind and these two aspects are so interrelated that they cannot be separated from one another.'

A large number of psychological manifestations have been described as the presenting features in various disorders, such as:

- Fainting
- Vertigo
- Delusion
- Stupor
- Anger
- Sorrow/remorse
- Anxiety
- Frustration
- Depression
- Mental fatigue

It is not possible to discuss all mental disorders in this chapter, so a few of the more common ones that can be treated relatively easily are discussed.

above **AYURVEDIC TREATMENT OF MENTAL ILLNESS OF ANY KIND IS A TREATMENT OF BOTH MIND AND BODY. THE CAUSE OF THE DISEASE MUST BE REMOVED AS WELL AS THE DISEASE ITSELF**

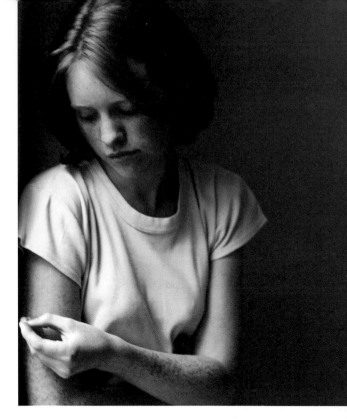

Case study: stress/anxiety

Davina Hamilton is a senior accounts executive in an advertising agency. Her work is extremely demanding and having to meet constant deadlines for both clients and the media, as well as her superiors, very often puts her in the firing line. Late nights and partying without adequate rest or irregular meals made her more tense and irritable.

She came to the Ayurvedic Hospital to find ways of relaxing and enjoying life, rather than suffering this constant tension. After a long consultation, the physician found her to have a pitta-vata constitution, which made it very difficult for her to relax. Davina had to learn to:

- Delegate work
- Be less competitive
- Take more time off from work
- Restrict late nights and meaningless parties
- Perform yoga and meditation
- Improve her diet to take in fresh vegetables, milk and butter
- Have shirodhara and massage
- Find a sympathetic soul mate

Two months after following this advice, Davina's life had totally changed. She is now a much more relaxed and gentler person who is aware that life is not simply about targets and client accounts.

MEMORY IMPAIRMENT

Chronic generalized reactions – including the loss of general intelligence, memory impairment, personality change and emotional changes – are collectively discussed under the term *dementia*. This is defined as a clinical syndrome characterized by a loss of previously acquired intellectual function in the absence of impaired consciousness.

Memory impairment can range from basic forgetfulness to the severity of Alzheimer's disease.

Case study: depression

Tessa Symons worked in a rather boring government department with a daily grind of files to push through the system. She lived with her elderly mother in a typical middle-class suburb with its attendant jealousies and pettiness, all of which alienated her sensitive soul even further. Her only love had long left her, knowing her dedication to her elderly mother was stronger than her feelings for him.

As she grew older, the days grew more and more gloomy, until one day she decided that she just did not want to live any more. She started thinking and even talking of suicide. At this stage, an old school friend advised her to see a therapist, as she thought it was a form of depression. A psychiatrist she saw at her friend's insistence analysed the cause as depression and gave her a mild 'mood-elevating' drug and told her to 'get on' with her life by 'getting a boyfriend' and taking holidays without her mother.

Tessa, however, had no intention of taking the addictive drug prescribed to her and went instead to see an ayurvedic practitioner. This doctor had a wiser and more spiritual understanding of her life and an appreciation of her duty to her mother. He explained that it was her 'karma' to fulfil this particular duty, but also indicated how she could take care of her mother and improve her own life if she were happier.

She was prescribed shirodhara, yoga and meditation, which she found to be extremely useful and 'mood elevating' without the need to resort to drugs. The yoga and medication helped her to have a happier attitude towards life and also to spend time away from home with other people. In fact, at her yoga class, she finally met and fell in love with a man to whom she eventually became engaged.

What are the symptoms?

The first sign of memory impairment is a minor degree of forgetfulness and short-term memory loss. Declining memory may lead to secondary delusions. In ayurveda, this is termed *smritinasa* or *smriti bhrama*, and is present in a number of disorders (as a warning symptom or a symptom in itself).

What is the treatment?

- Brahmi ghrita – 10 g twice daily
- Saraswata choornam – 3 g two or three times a day
- Saraswatarishta – 30 ml twice daily
- Shankhapushpi syrup – 2 teaspoons three times daily
- Brahmi taila – to be massaged into the scalp
- Bhringaraj taila – to be massaged into the scalp

ANXIETY AND DEPRESSION

Anxiety and depression – universal experiences – are the result of reactions to certain situational challenges and form an essential response system to the environment. Both these reactions serve a useful purpose when the response is within an 'acceptable' range and is said to be normal – although there is no clear distinction between the features of normal and pathological anxiety. An exaggerated response either in degree or duration, that is, when symptoms are out of proportion or they persist long after a threatening situation has been averted, certainly affects the social, physiological and psychological functioning and is considered detrimental to your health. This level of either anxiety or depression is pathological and needs to be corrected by either a drug or a non-drug therapy.

Symptoms of anxiety are present in other psychiatric disorders such as schizophrenia and depressive illnesses. There are several physical illnesses which can also present with anxiety. In ayurveda, a number of physical illnesses, as well as psychiatric illnesses, present with symptoms of anxiety and depression, and the treatment involves the use of ayurvedic drugs, relaxation techniques and panchakarma, including shirodhara.

What causes anxiety and depression?

According to ayurveda, depression is caused by both karmic imbalances and either aggravated vata or kapha, or both. Excessive kapha that causes weight gain can cause lethargy and depression, whereas exacerbated vata can cause insecurity, anxiety or depression. Other causes are:

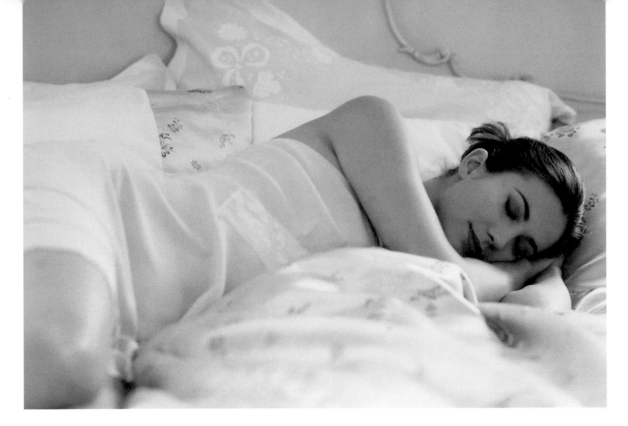

- Broken relationships
- Grief and shock
- Death of a loved one
- Poverty
- Unemployment
- Illness
- Incurable disease

What are the symptoms?

- Disturbed sleep, such as insomnia or oversleeping
- Lack of energy
- Loss of appetite and weight
- Overeating and weight gain
- Lack of concentration
- Feelings of hopelessness
- Disinterest in friends and usual activities

What is the treatment?

Key aspects of the treatment of anxiety and depression are explanation and reassurance. If you do not respond to these, relaxation techniques may be prescribed. Shirodhara, yoga and meditation are also used. It is important to realize that clinical depression is a serious illness, so qualified advice should always be sought.

AYURVEDIC MEDICINES
- Aswagandha choornam – 3–6 g in milk once or twice a day
- Aswagandharishta – 30 ml twice daily
- Brahmi svasasa – 5 ml twice daily
- Saraswatarishtam – 20 ml twice daily
- Brahma rasayana – 3–6 g twice daily
- Brahmi ghrita – 10 g twice daily

Insomnia

Insomnia (*adindra*) is a condition where a person complains of inadequate or poor-quality sleep due to a combination of factors, including underlying physical or mental disorders. It is not defined by the number of hours of sleep a person gets or how long it takes to fall asleep. The need for sleep and its satisfaction vary from person to person. Lack of sleep at night can cause problems during the day, such as fatigue, lack of energy, difficulty concentrating and irritability.

Insomnia can be classified as transient (short term), intermittent (occasional) or chronic (constant). When it lasts from a single night to a few weeks it is referred to as transient. If transient insomnia occurs from time to time, it is considered intermittent; if it occurs on most nights and lasts a month or more, it is termed chronic.

Chronic insomnia is a complex condition, the most common cause of which is depression. Other disorders presenting with insomnia are arthritis, heart disease, asthma, restless leg syndrome and sleep apnoea.

above **AYURVEDA IDENTIFIES AND REMOVES THE CAUSE OF INSOMNIA, WHILE TREATMENTS SUCH AS SHIRODHARA, COMBINE WELL WITH YOGA AND MEDITATION TO RELIEVE THE SYMPTOMS**

Other general causes include:

- Stress
- Environmental noise
- Extreme temperatures
- Change in surrounding environment
- Medication side effects
- Misuse of caffeine, alcohol and other substances
- Napping in the afternoon or evening

What is the treatment?

Ayurveda's time-tested approach to treatment – remove the cause and the effect will disappear – works well with insomnia. Diagnosing the underlying cause and treating any medical and psychological problems will help you to overcome this problem.

Methods of treatment include:

- Shirodhara
- Yoga and meditation
- Relaxation therapy to reduce anxiety and tension

AYURVEDIC MEDICINES
- Aswangandha choornam – 3–6 g twice daily
- Aswagandharishta – 20 ml twice daily
- Nidrodaya rasa – 120 mg once in the evening
- Saraswata choornam – 3 g twice daily with honey
- Brahmi taila – to massage on the head/scalp

Prognosis

Insomnia is very easily treated in ayurveda, particularly with the use of shirodhara, yoga and meditation.

Diseases of the bones and joints

Bones provide the structural support to our body and its components, and help to keep the body upright. Another vital, but not so obvious, role of bones is to act like 'girders' to which muscles are attached. Bones are hollow inside, and the body, with great economy of space, uses these cavities for the manufacture of blood cells from the marrow in the bone's cavity. Bones also manufacture another vital substance, calcium.

The cells of the bone produce fibrous tissue, a relatively soft and pliable 'base' material upon which is built a network of harder material that provides strength; the end product is an extremely strong structure with considerable flexibility.

Bones start forming in the human body during the first month of pregnancy. At this stage, they resemble cartilage tissue (soft material with a rubber-like flexibility). As the foetus grows, this cartilage frame is replaced by fibrous tissue. Hardening of the bones is a gradual process that takes place throughout childhood and is only completed by the end of puberty. The bones are connected by joints. The ends of the bones are covered with a pad of soft cartilage so that during movement and weight bearing they do not damage each other. The joint is also lubricated by a fluid known as synovial fluid, formed inside the synovial cavity, that is surrounded by synovial membrane. The whole structure of the joints is tied together by tough tissues known as ligaments.

Bones have the extraordinary ability to maintain their structure when infected or injured. The most obvious example of this is their ability to repair themselves, even when broken or cracked.

The ayurvedic view

Bone tissue is known as *asthi dhatu* in ayurveda, and it is one of the seven tissues of the body. Bone is termed *asthi*, while a joint is called *sandhi*. Our bones are considered to be the hardest tissue in the body. They are formed mainly from the basic elements of earth

below **MASSAGE USING SPECIAL AYURVEDIC OILS HELPS TO MANIPULATE THE JOINTS AND REJUVENATE THE CHANNELS OF THE BODY TO RELIEVE BONE DISORDERS**

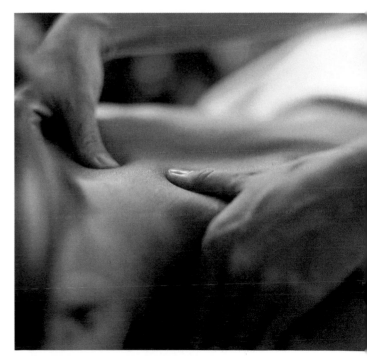

and air; the air element being dominant in the central marrow cavity. Earth and air elements in the body are carried by rasa (plasma) and rakta (blood), and brought together by kapha at the site of bone formation. The digestive enzymes in the bony tissue – the epiphyseal or periosteal cartilage (*asthi agni*) – digest solid, air and 'kapha' elements, as well as essential nutrients from fatty tissue, thereby synthesizing bone.

What is the treatment?

Generally, all disorders of the bones and joints are treated in the same manner, following the principles for correction of the bone channels of the body. Treatment includes panchakarma, particularly enema therapy (*basti*) using an enema of milk and ghee processed with bitter herbs.

Guggulu (a gum resin obtained from the plant *Comiphora mukul*) and shilajit (an extract from rocks) are excellent substances for the treatment of various bone problems. In ayurvedic practice, doctors use various compounds derived from guggulu, such as yogaraja guggulu, trayoda sharya guggulu, rasnadi guggulu and chandrapraba vati. Garlic is also very beneficial for bone diseases, particularly those arising from metabolic disorders, as well as bone fractures.

Massage with oils such as balaswagandhadi taila, lakshadi taila and pinda taila are extremely useful in relieving many bone disorders.

Excellent sources of calcium and other minerals required for remodelling of fractured bones which are derived from various mineral sources and animal bones, include: shankha bhasma, kukkutaanda twak bhasma, mouktika bhasma and mriga shringa bhasma.

Guggulu tikta kashayam and guggulu tikta ghrita are the ayurvedic medicines of choice for bone disorders.·

Your diet should mainly consist of wheat, black gram, radish, beetroot, sugar cane, dates, garlic, ginger, milk and ghee (clarified butter).

RHEUMATOID ARTHRITIS

Rheumatoid arthritis is a disease that mainly affects the joints, but may, in severe cases, affect other organs, such as the heart, lungs, nervous system and the eyes. It occurs in both men and women, but is more prevalent in females. It is a chronic condition that is frequently punctuated by periods when, for no apparent reason, the symptoms become worse,

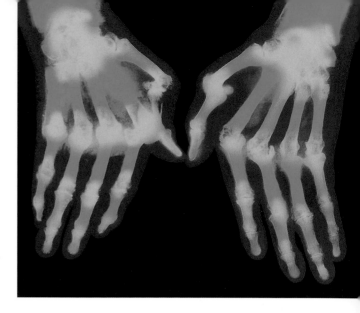

above and right **AN EFFECTIVE TREATMENT FOR RHEUMATOID ARTHRITIS IS BALWKA SWEDA, A GRAIN-FILLED POULTICE WHICH IS DIPPED IN OIL, HEATED AND APPLIED TO THE PAINFUL AREA**

lessen or disappear. It can sometimes occur in children aged between two and three years and may progress throughout their life, leading to deformities.

The basic cause of rheumatoid arthritis is not still clear. The disease occurs when the body's immune system reacts to the presence of the initiating agent and tries to eliminate it. This immune response causes an accumulation of inflamed cells within the synovial membrane – the inner lining of cavities of joints and sheaths of tendons that secrete the synovial fluid.

The ayurvedic view

All types of rheumatism are manifestations of a vata imbalance, according to ayurveda. *Amavata* and *vatarakta*, two diseases described in ayurvedic texts, are very similar to rheumatoid arthritis and gouty arthritis.

What causes rheumatoid arthritis?

Rheumatism is caused by routine indulgence in foods that are incompatible, by people with very weak or poor agni (digestive fire), and who basically lead a sedentary lifestyle. Rheumatism also afflicts people who consume a fatty diet and do not get enough exercise.

When food is not digested properly, undigested material, ama (toxins or metabolic waste), forms. This becomes associated with the doshas and, as a result, creates diseases of various kinds. Amavata (rheumatoid arthritis) is caused by unwholesome dietary habits. In amavata, the ama links up with vata and, because of the nature of vata, is carried to various joints of the body. Here it becomes lodged and gives rise to a variety of symptoms including joint pain, swelling and stiffness.

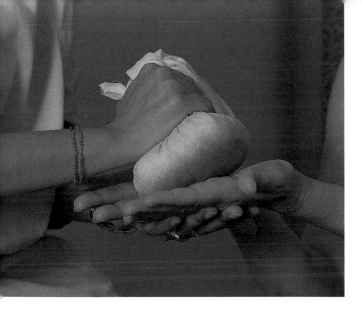

In vatarakta (gouty arthritis), both incompatible foods and activities cause vata and rakta (blood) to become unbalanced, giving rise to symptoms of pain, swelling of joints and rashes over the skin. In this condition, pitta- and vata-balancing remedies are indicated.

Pathology

The causes listed above usually help to accumulate ama (a product of digestion and metabolism – free radicals). The unbalanced vayu (air) carries this ama to various centres affected by vata, pitta and kapha. Here it putrefies and produces an obstruction to the channels of body fluids. This further affects agni (digestive fire), producing increased ama, and hence a vicious cycle develops. Ama is capable of manifesting as several diseases and is of a very serious nature.

In rheumatoid arthritis, vayu (air) and kapha, both afflicted by ama, enter the joints and make them stiff, tender and swollen.

What are the symptoms?

- Mild fever and generalized aches and pains at onset
- Sudden development of joint inflammation
- Swollen joints
- Red, warm, painful joints
- Stiffness which is more severe in the morning
- Weak grip
- Raynaud's phenomenon (fingers turn bluish-white on exposure to cold)
- Soft nodules beneath the skin
- Bursitis (fluid-filled sac around the joints)
- Baker's cyst (fluid-filled swelling behind the knee joint)
- Fatigue followed by anaemia
- Deformity of joints in the later stages of the disease

Rheumatoid arthritis is understood to be the most painful of all diseases. When ama is removed from the joint, the symptoms disappear.

If pitta dominates the pathology, there will be an increase in the burning sensation and redness. If vata is the main dosha involved, the pain is severe. If kapha dominates, heaviness, itching and a sensation of being covered with a wet cloth predominate.

This disease can also give rise to many other complications, such as loss of digestive power (agni), excessive salivation, anorexia, heaviness, loss of enthusiasm, an unpleasant taste in the mouth, a burning sensation in the body, sleep disturbances, thirst, vomiting, giddiness and fainting, chest pain, constipation and speech disorders.

What is the treatment?

The main principle in the treatment of rheumatoid arthritis is to increase agni (fire) and digest ama. The removal of ama is the first and most important step. Herbs are then prescribed to balance vata and kapha.

Case study: rheumatoid arthritis

Jenny Bolton is a woman in her fifties who suffers from rheumatoid arthritis. She had had the illness for more than four years and did not get any relief at all from her doctor's prescription of, at first, painkillers and later, steroids. The pain and the swellings on her hands and knees kept increasing over the years and she began feeling the side effects of taking steroids, such as the classic 'moon face' (round, heavy face), osteoporosis and thinning of the skin.

In desperation, she came to the Ayurvedic Charitable Hospital for treatment, where she was prescribed:

- Massage and herbal sauna
- Herbal enema
- Application of herbal poultices
- Guggulu as internal medication

The massage, sauna and poultices immediately reduced the pain and swelling, and, after three herbal enemas, Jenny's pain had completely disappeared. In fact, she lost almost 5 kg (11 lbs) of excess weight and is now looking radiantly healthy and free of the problems caused by her rheumatoid arthritis. A year later, she has had no remissions of her illness.

Treatment for rheumatoid arthritis mainly consists of oil massage, herbal sauna and basti (medicated enema). If ama symptoms are observed, herbal drugs to digest ama such as trikatu, ginger and panchakola are prescribed. In chronic cases of rheumatoid arthritis, detoxification and cleansing of the body with panchakarma are recommended.

Castor oil is the best remedy for rheumatism, and it should be taken by mixing it with a decoction of dashamoola (ten root herbs) and ginger.

Useful herbs include: eranda (*Ricinus communis*), rasna (*Pluchea lanceolata*), dasamool, guggulu (*Commiphora mukul*) and yogaraj guggulu. Guduchi (*Tinospora cordifolia*) is another useful herb for relief from rheumatism, if taken with ginger.

A number of formulations are available in ayurveda, such as rasnadashamool kashayam, rasnapanchaka kashayam, eranda haritaki, vaishvanara choornam, saindhavadi taila, vishnu taila, yogaraj guggulu, simhanad guggulu and kasona sura. However, they should be used only after consulting a qualified ayurvedic physician.

If you suffer from rheumatoid arthritis, you should avoid yogurt, fish, jaggery (palm sugar), milk, black gram, pastries and other foods that are heavy to digest and which obstruct the body's channels of circulation (*abhishyandhi*).

Prognosis

Rheumatoid arthritis is very difficult to cure, but symptoms can be relieved during treatment. Ayurvedic treatment may prevent deformity and complications if carried out regularly for five to six months, and if dietary and lifestyle recommendations are followed strictly once treatment is complete.

OSTEOARTHRITIS

Osteoarthritis is a common disease afflicting the joints which is aggravated by mechanical stress. It is characterized by degeneration of the cartilage that lines joints, or by formation of bony outgrowths (osteophytes) which lead to pain, stiffness and occasionally loss of function of the affected joint.

Osteoarthritis occurs in almost all people aged over 60, although not all exhibit symptoms. Various factors lead to the development of osteoarthritis earlier in life, including an injury to a joint or a congenital joint deformity. Three times as many women as men are affected by this ailment. Although any joint can show osteoarthritic changes, the knees and the spine are the most commonly affected.

The ayurvedic view

Arthritis is considered in ayurvedic medicine as *sandhi vata* or *sandhiasthigata vata*. Basically, it is a disorder associated with vata imbalance in the body.

Vata is the counterpart of the universal element of vayu (air), which is life, strength and the sustainer of creatures. Vata is the principle that operates the movements in our bodies. Our bones and joints are bodily nuts and bolts which enable us to move freely. They are the seat of vata in the body. Any imbalance in vata may result in discomfort to the bone or joint, and thus restrict your movement.

When the five kinds of vayu operating in our body are in equilibrium and located in their rightful place, they perform their normal functions so that the body is free of disorders. If they are displaced or unbalanced, they afflict the body with disorders relating to their location and functions, thus removing the pleasure of life. Although the disorders caused by vata are innumerable, the most important ones, numbering approximately 80, have been described extensively in ayurvedic literature.

Unbalanced vata usually produces contractions, stiffness in joints, tearing in bones and joints, goose flesh or goose bumps, delirium, stiffness in the hands, back and head, limping, crippling pain and deformity, drying of organs, sleeplessness, distress, mental confusion and exhaustion. Pain is an important manifestation of vata imbalances, and it is a feature of all forms of arthritis.

What causes osteoarthritis?

All the factors that cause imbalance of vata are also the causes of arthritis. These include excessive movements such as leaping, jumping and physical exercise, an uncomfortable bed or seat, suppression of natural body urges, injury to the vital parts (*marma*), falling from vehicles or animals, and foods that are rough, cold and eaten in small quantities.

The various causes of arthritis usually aggravate vata, which fills the body's vacant channels, ducts and spaces, thereby producing various disorders, including arthritis to one or several parts of the body (for example, either a single or several joints).

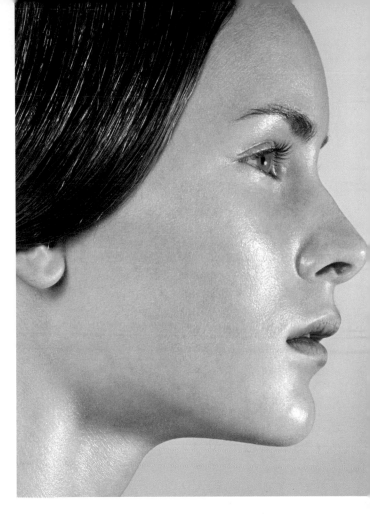

right SEEKING PROPER AYURVEDIC TREATMENT FOR COMMON AND NOT-SO-COMMON AILMENTS CAN TRANSFORM YOUR LIFE. THE BENEFITS FOR YOUR HEALTH AND WELLBEING CAN BE MANIFOLD WHETHER THEY ARE PHYSICAL, MENTAL OR SPIRITUAL

What are the symptoms?

- Pain, stiffness, swelling or cracking of one or more joints
- Weakness and shrinkage of surrounding muscle
- Enlargement of affected joint
- Deformed joints in some cases

What is the treatment?

The treatment of osteoarthritis is generally based on a principle of balancing vata. It can be performed through external physical therapy, internal purification (*panchakarma*), vata-balancing diets, drugs and herbs.

When there is pain, swelling and stiffness in the joint, it is advisable to apply external manipulation of the joint using oils such as marmani taila, kottamchukkadi taila and pinda taila.

This should be followed by different types of sweating therapy (*swedana*) using steam, dry heat and heat oil gram bolus (*pinda sweda*). You may also be advised to use herbs and processed medicated oils, such as bala taila, dhanwantaram taila, sahacharadi taila and ksheerabala taila.

A course of herbal and medicated oil enema therapy (*basti*) is very useful in all types of arthritis. Therefore, oil therapy (*snehana*) with oil and ghee, and sweating therapy (*swedana*) form the basis of treatment. This can be supported by enema therapy (*basti*) and mild purgatives using avipathikara choornam, gandharva hastadi, eranda taila and so on.

Your diet should mainly consist of sour gruels, soups made from meat, marrow and sour substances, sweet porridges and milk puddings. Kitchari a therapeutic food made of rice and moong dal with some mild spices – is also advised (see page 101). You should avoid over-exercise and repetitive strain, such as jogging or high-impact aerobics.

External application of medicated oils and herbal pastes and poultices is also used. Occasionally potions made of dashanga, atasyadi or shothagee applied over the affected joint help to relieve swelling and pain immediately. Hot oil can also be poured over the affected joint. Oils such as dhanwantaram taila and bala taila are recommended.

Some formulations based on guggulu (a gum from the plant *Commiphora mukul*) are very useful as prescription drugs. The different kinds of guggulu preparations available in ayurveda include yogaraja guggulu, trayodashanga guggulu, saptavimshati guggulu and kaishore guggulu.

Various herbal decoctions such as dasamoolam kashayam, maharasnadi kashayam, rasna saptaka quath, rasna erandadi kashayam, sahacharadi kashayam and prarasenyadi kashayam are also useful in the treatment of osteoarthritis.

Herb and mineral preparations such as mahavata vidwamsa ras and bhosla vajrin ras are very effective in giving immediate relief.

A final note

Remember, ayurvedic preparations should be prescribed only by a qualified ayurvedic doctor. The dose, duration of treatment, any dietary restrictions and so on should always be followed. Each treatment is tailored to the prakruti (physical constitution) of the individual patient and the specific underlying cause.

glossary

agni – internal fire or digestive capacity (metabolism). There are three main types: jatharagni, bhootagni and dhatwagni.

akasha – space, or ether (one of the five basic elements of the universe)

ama – toxic material (e.g. undigested food), the root cause of ill health

annavaha srotas – the channels of the digestive system

ap – water (one of the five basic elements of the universe)

asthi – hard tissues (mainly bones)

atma – your true self or soul

ayurvedic massage – there are several forms of massage used in ayurveda, including abhyanga (for vata, pitta and kapha constitutions), padabhyanga (foot massage) and dry (seasonal) massage

ayurvedic medicines – these are based on five formulations: swarasa (the expressed juice of a plant), kalka (paste), kashaya (decoction), choornam (powder) and vati or gutika (tablet or pill)

basti – the administration of medicated enemas. Used for almost all diseases, but mainly for vata disorders and rejuvenation. There are three types: aphrodisiac, oil and decoction.

body tissues – the seven tissues of rasa (plasma), rakta (blood), mamsa (muscular tissue), meda (fatty tissue), asthi (bone), maija (marrow and nerve tissue) and shukra (reproductive tissue)

Brahma – the Hindu god Lord Brahma is seen as the creator of the universe and the original proponent of ayurveda

buddhi – intellect

chakra – meaning 'wheel', part of the principle of kundalini, these are the body's centres of spiritual energy

Charaka Samhita – classic ayurvedic text on internal medicine

chikitsa – a method or procedure which brings about equilibrium in the body's doshas, tissues, waste products, etc.

dharma – moral path

dhatu – body tissues

dhyana – meditation

dinacharya – daily regimen

dosha – body humour. There are three doshas: vata, pitta and kapha. They are responsible for all physiological actions in the body

gem therapy – treatment with precious stones to help reduce the impact of planetary afflictions

guna – attribute

Kali – goddess of destruction

kapha – one of the three doshas

karma – the law of action

kitchari – a dish made from mung beans, often prescribed as part of a therapeutic diet

kundalini – energy of the subtle or astral body, the spiritual life force

langhana – purifying treatment or procedure which brings lightness in the body

maija – nerve tissue and bone marrow

mala – waste product of the body, i.e. faeces, urine or perspiration

mamsa – muscular tissue

marma – any one of 107 vital energy points in the body

meda – fatty tissue

nasya – a medicine through the nasal route

panchakarma – the five purification therapies: vamana (emesis), virechana (purgation), basti (enema), nasya (nasal) and raktamoksha (blood letting)

panchamahabhutas – the five basic elements of the universe: air, space, water, fire and earth

pathogenesis – the process of a disease's manifestation

pitta – one of the three doshas

poorva karma – treatment regime undertaken before panchakarma

prabhava – the strength or special effects of a certain medium (e.g. the actions of particular herbs)

prajnaparadha – action against consciousness/morality

prakruti – physical nature or constitution

prana – breath of life

pranayama – type of yoga

pratyaksha – the direct observation of objects

prithyi – earth (one of the five basic elements of the universe)

prodormal – the primary stage of disease manifestation

rajas – one of the three gunas which forms our mental or psychological constitution. Rajas is typefied by mixed qualities or human traits

rakta – blood, which maintains life

raktamoksha – blood letting

rasa – means either plasma (as in rasa dhatu) or taste. There are six tastes: sweet (madhura), sour (amla), salty (katu), pungent (lavana), bitter (tikta) and astringent (kashayam)

rasayana – rejuvenation therapy aimed at improving strength and vitality, immunity against disease and longevity

ritucharya – seasonal regimen

rukshana – drying

satwa – mind

satwic – one of the three gunas which forms our mental or psychological constitution. Satwic represents the good qualities of mind, a pure and noble person

shadrasas – the six tastes

shirodhara – pouring of warm medicated oil on the forehead

Shiva – Lord Shiva, Hindu god of creation and destruction

shukra – semen, reproductive tissue

snehana – oil therapy (both internal and external)

srota – channel

sthambhana – stopping (blocking)

Sushruta Samhita – an ayurvedic text which deals mainly with surgery

swedana – sweating therapy

tamas – one of the three gunas which forms our mental or psychological constitution. Tamas represents id, or the lower or base tendencies of human nature

tanmatra – shabda (sound), sparsha (touch), roopa (vision), rasa (touch) and ganda (smell)

teja – fire (one of the five basic elements of the universe)

upadhatus – the subtissues and main tissues of the body

Upanishad – classical philosophical texts which form part of the Vedas

upasthambha – the pillars of life: dhara (food), nidra (sleep) and Brahmacharya (sex and spirituality)

vamana – emesis therapy

vastu shastra – Indian science of improving the benevolent energies of houses and property, which is somewhat similar to feng shui

vata – one of the three doshas

vayu – air (one of the five basic elements of the universe)

Vedas – ancient Indian scriptures, including Ayur Veda, Yajur Veda, Sama Veda and Athara Veda

veerya – potency

vipaka – end product of food

virechana – purgation therapy

virilification therapy – rejuvenation therapy designed to improve virility and fertility

Vishnu – a name for God in Hinduism

yoga – the uniting of the mind and the body, and the energies within

further reading directory

Frawley, David, *Ayurveda and the Mind: The Healing of Consciousness*, Motilal Banarsidass Publishers, New Delhi, 1998.

Tiwari, Maya, *Ayurveda: A Life of Balance*, Healing Arts Press, Rochester, USA, 1995.

Svoboda, Robert E., *Prakruti: Your Ayurvedic Constitution*, Geocom Press, Albuquerque, NM, 1988.

Bhagwan Dash, *Basic Principles of Ayurveda*, Concept Publishing Co., New Delhi, 1980

Lad, Vasant, *Ayurveda, the Science of Self-Healing: A Practical Guide*, Lotus Press, Santa Fe, NM 1984.

Sharma, P. V., *Charaka Samhita, Sutrasthanam*, vol. I, Chaukhambha Orientalia, Varanasi, India, 1996.

Udupa, K. N. & Singh, R. H. (eds), *Science of Philosophy of Indian Medicine*, Sree Baidyanath Ayurveda Bhawan Ltd, Nagpur, India, 1978.

Gerson, Scott, MD, *Health Essentials: Ayurveda - The Ancient Indian Healing Art*, Element, Rockport, MA, 1993.

Bhishagratna, K. L. (trans.), *Sushrata Samhita*, Sanskrit series, Chaukhambha, Varanasi, India, 1981.

Frawley, David & Lad, Vasant, *The Yoga of Herbs: An Ayurvedic Guide to Herbal Medicine*, Lotus Press, Santa Fe, NM, 1988.

Srikantha Murthy, Prof. K. R., *Madhava Nidanam (Roga Viniscaya) of Madhavakara: A Treatise on Ayurveda*, Jaikrishnadas Ayurveda Series, no. 69, Chaukhambha Orientalia, New Delhi, 1987.

Bhagwan Dash, Vaidya & Junuis, Acarya Manfred M., *A Handbook of Ayurveda*, Concept Publishing Co., New Delhi, 1983.

Srikantha Murthy, Prof. K. R., *Doctrines of Pathology in Ayurveda*, Vidyavilas Ayurveda Series, no. 3, Chaukhambha Prietalia, Varansani, India, 1987.

Shiv Sharma, Pandit, *Ayurvedic Medicine, Past and Present*, Dabur Publications, Calcutta, 1975.

The Potential for Herbal Medicines in the World Pharmaceutical Industry, McAlpine, Thorpe & Warrier Limited, London, 1988.

Who's Who in the World Herbal Medical Industry, McAlpine, Thorpe & Warrier Limited, London, 1995.

Kinsley, David, *Hindu Goddesses: Visions of the Divine Feminine in the Hindu Religious Tradition*, Motilal Banarsidass, New Delhi.

Kinsley, David, *The Divine Player*, Motilal Banaridass.

Majumdar, R. C., Rachaudhuri, H. C. & Datta, Kalikinkar, *An Advanced History of India*, St. Martin's Press, New York, 1967.

The Siva-Purana (trans.), 4 vols, Motilal Banarsidass, Delhi, 1970.

Nataraja in Art, Thought and Literature, National Museum, New Delhi, 1974.

Wilson, H. H. (trans.), *The Vishnu Purana: A System of Hindu Mythology and Tradition*, Punthi Pushtak, Calcutta, 1961.

Warrier, Gopi & Gunawant, Deepika, MD, *The Complete Illustrated Guide to Ayurveda*, Element Books, Rockport, MA, 1997.

Warrier, Gopi & Verma, Dr H., *Secrets of Ayurveda*, Dorling Kindersley, London, 2001.

AYURVEDIC COLLEGES

Ayurvedic Company of Great Britain
81 Wimpole Street
London W1G 9RF, England
www.unifiedherbal.com

Arya Vaidya Pharmacy
1382 Trichy Road
Coimbatore 641018
South India

Arya Vaidya Sala Hospital
Kottakkal 676503
Dist:Mallapuram
Kerala State
South India

Faculty of Ayurveda Institute of Medical Sciences
Benaras Hindu University
Varanasi 221005, India

WESTERN AYURVEDIC & HERBAL INSTITUTIONS

American Institute of Vedic Studies
P O Box 8357
Santa Fe, NM 87504
USA

The Ayurvedic Company of Great Britain Ltd
81 Wimpole Street
London W1G 9RF, England
www.unifiedherbal.com

The Ayurvedic Institute
P O Box 282
Fairfield, IA 52556
USA

The Ayurvedic Institute of Wellness Center
1131 Menual N.E.
Albuquerque, NM 87112
USA

Maharishi Ayurveda
579 Punt Road
South Yarra VIC 3141
Australia

AYURVEDIC THERAPY CENTRES AND SPAS

Arya Vaidya Sala Hospital
Kottakkal 676503
Dist: Mallapuram
Kerala State
South India

The Ayurvedic Charitable Hospital
47 Nottingham Place
London W1, England

The Ayurvedic Therapy Clinic
81 Wimpole Street
London W1G 9RF, England

Heythrop Park
Contact: 81 Wimpole Street
London W1G 9RF, England

ASSOCIATIONS

Academie International des Medecines Naturelles
52 Boulevard Flandrin
75116 Paris, France

American Association of Ayurvedic Medicine
PO Box 598
South Lancaster
MA 01561, USA

American Herbal Products Association
8484 Georgia Avenue
Suite 370
Silver Spring, MD 20910
USA

American Holistic Medical Association
4101 Lake Boone Trail,
Suite 201, Raleigh,
North Carolina 27607, USA

British Association of Accredited Ayurvedic Practitioners
64 Gloucester Road
Kew, Richmond
Surrey TW9 3BX
England

British Ayurvedic Medical Council
47 Nottingham Place
London W1, England

Council for Complementary and Alternative Medicine
19a Cavendish Square
London W1M 9AD
England

Economic Botany Symposium
New York Botanical Gardens
Bronx, NY 10458
USA

index

PICTURE CREDITS
The publishers would like to thank the following sources for their kind permission to reproduce the pictures in this book:

Art Archive: 8, 10 / Ayurvedic Company of Great Britain: 1, 82, 83t, 83b, 121 / Carlton Books: 2–3, 11, 31t, 31c, 31br, 37tr, 37tm, 37c, 37br, 57, 58, 62, 67, 73, 76, 79, 91, 119 / David Garcia: 52 / Getty Images Imagebank: 4–5, 30, 40, 85 / Getty Images Stone: 13, 14 from top down, 24, 37tr, 44, 66, 71, 80, 87 / Getty Images Telegraph: 30, 92 / Robert Harding: 53, 68 / Alex Sarginson: 16, 54 / Science Photo Library: 23, 89, 94, 104 / Jim Spelman: 123

ACKNOWLEDGEMENTS
The author gratefully acknowledges the help of the following people: David McAlpine for photographs of vata, pitta and kapha types; Lady Morrit for photographs; Dr Hadapad for glossary; and Kamla Jassal for typing services.